The Baldness Cure

The Baldness Cure

The Unique Regrowth Programme that Really Works

Andy Bryant

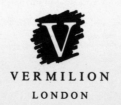

VERMILION

LONDON

First published 1994

3 5 7 9 10 8 6 4

Text & photographs © Natural Hair Marketing Ltd 1994

First published in the United Kingdom in 1994 by
Vermilion
an imprint of Ebury Press
Random House, 20 Vauxhall Bridge Road, London SWIV 2SA

Random House Australia (Pty) Limited
20 Alfred Street, Milsons Point, Sydney,
New South Wales 2061, Australia

Random House New Zealand Limited
18 Poland Road, Glenfield,
Auckland 10, New Zealand

Random House South Africa (Pty) Limited
PO Box 337, Bergvlei, South Africa

Random House UK Limited Reg. No. 954009

A CIP catalogue record for this book is available from the British Library

ISBN: 0 09 178242 2

Typeset in 11.5/13.5, Baskerville by
Pure Tech Corporation, Pondicherry, India
Printed and bound in Great Britain by Mackays of Chatham Plc, Kent

Papers used by Ebury Press are natural, recyclable products made from wood grown in sustainable forests.

Front cover photographs: These two photographs show the progress made by David Clark-Wilson between April 1992 (LH photo) and November 1993 (RH photo). The size of his bald area has been reduced from 102 sq cm to 20 sq cm (80% reduction) and his hair continues to grow.

*This book is dedicated to Mervyn Minall-Jones,
who taught me the true meaning of the word intuition*

Contents

Introduction

One evening in May 1992 my telephone rang. It was a friend of mine called David, sounding very excited: 'It worked, we must meet tonight and plan it all.'

Before I could ask what he was talking about, he said: 'I am growing my hair back using your programme, although I have been partly bald for ten years.'

David had managed to do what I had also done: reversed the process of going bald.

That evening, we discussed a plan to experiment with another one hundred people, just to make sure we were not freaks, and included some women in our sample, too. Well over ninety per cent of these people began to reverse their baldness within four months, so we kept expanding the numbers.

As I sit here writing this book, letter after letter, telephone call after telephone call confirms that I have solved the age-old mystery of why we go bald and how to reverse it. The basis of my success and that of so many others is following a carefully planned programme for hair growth. That programme is outlined in the following chapters of *The Baldness Cure*.

The medical profession has largely narrowed down the cause of baldness to the effect of the male hormone testosterone.

Their belief is that testosterone directly affects the root of the hair and stops it growing, although this belief is now disputed by some doctors. The world has been awaiting a wonder drug that will act like a little net around the base of the hair follicle and stop the testosterone getting through.

In my search to solve my own hair-loss problem, I was amazed at the ridiculous solutions offered to me. These included 'paddy fields' in the form of transplants that would come out of the back of my head; drugs that were originally designed to reduce high blood pressure; and all sorts of potions and lotions. The final straw was when I was offered female hormones!

I discovered that the direct effect of testosterone on the hair follicle could be ignored; however, its overall effect on the body could be observed to be producing baldness. The importance of this discovery was that I could reverse the effects testosterone was having, so demonstrating that I was correct, and could re-grow lost hair. Having reversed the balding process, I could then teach people what the real cause was and deal with that too. At last I could help people grow their hair back in a natural way, without drugs.

What I was not prepared for was the improvements in the general health of those following the programme. Do not be surprised if you too find that your overall health benefits while you are on the programme.

The programme is not a magic cure – just believe that by following it, as I and many others have done, you too can restore your lost hair growth. Let this book be your guide on the road to success.

Basic facts about hair

Our hair protects our heads from the sun and from injury. The part we can see above the surface is the hairshaft, with the root below the skin's surface. Figure 1 outlines the structure that exists below the skin.

The hairshaft consists of dead cells, which is why a haircut is not painful. Each hair consists of cells that proliferate and manufacture keratin as they move outward and then die.

STRUCTURE OF A GROWING HAIR (Figure 1)

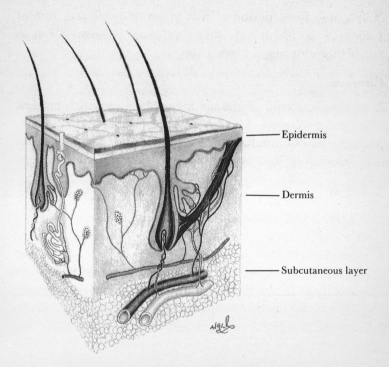

Epidermis

Dermis

Subcutaneous layer

Cycles of growth

The average head has about 100,000 hairs, of which ninety per cent are usually in the growing phase. The growing phase (anagen) is followed by a resting phase (telogen). After that a new hair grows in the same follicle, pushing the old one out. The period of change between is called catagen.

It follows that ten per cent of the hair can be resting at any one time; as this is not synchronized, up to ninety hairs a day can be lost in a naturally healthy head.

Anagen

Hair grows for a period of two to seven years at a rate of 1.25cm a month. It may therefore grow between 30cm to 1m before entering a resting stage.

Catagen

A two-week period of change takes place in which no new cells are produced. The lower part of the hair detaches from the base of the follicle to form a club hair. Only about one per cent of hair at a time enters this period of change.

Telogen

The resting phase lasts three to four months.

It is important that you stop worrying about losing hair from this moment forward. Through this book you will discover how to overcome baldness, although the changes you will make on the programme may take some time to work through. The hairs that you are currently losing are either being pushed out by new replacements or are due to damage, caused some time ago, that you can do nothing about. You can only change the *future* of your hair.

Blood supply to the skin

One of the skin's many important roles is to regulate our temperature. Heat is released as cells metabolize nutrients; this heat must be regulated to prevent our temperature from continually rising.

A complex blood supply to the skin is needed to keep our temperature at an optimum of 36.1°C to 37.8°C.

During rest, our skeletal muscles (see Chapter 2, p.38) are only responsible for twenty to thirty per cent of the body's heat, but this can rise to produce forty times more heat than the rest of the body.

Rapid changes in temperature are possible because of the alternative pathways for blood at different levels of the skin.

When you examine a head in an advanced state of baldness, it is apparent that the dermis has atrophied, whilst the epidermis is still intact. In simple terms the fleshiness has gone and the scalp feels woody.

The amount of blood in the surface of the skin is controlled by nerve endings in the artery walls. These receptors cause vasodilation or constriction, depending on their temperature, thereby increasing or reducing blood flow.

It is my hypothesis that whilst the blood supply to the follicle may be temporarily halted during stress, the skin's supply will need to be kept open for temperature control. If the constriction in the hair follicle continues for too long, it causes not only hair loss but also atrophy of the subcutaneous layer.

Why I began to investigate baldness

Like many men, by my late twenties I had already begun to recede considerably at the front of my head. My father had a considerable hair loss problem which progressed gradually throughout his life. While I had assumed that I too would lose my hair, I had not expected it to go so fast or for the loss to come in short rapid bouts followed by periods of no apparent loss.

Something puzzled me, though. My elder brother, nearly four years my senior, had a full head of hair, and my younger brother, four years my junior, seemed to be losing hair at a faster rate than me. If it were hereditary, why was there this variation amongst three brothers of the same parents?

Quite frankly, I hated it. Every morning I would see that the pillow was covered in hair, and the shower plug would regularly clog up stopping the water running away. I recalled that as a child I had had great difficulty combing my hair because it was so thick, and I had to use a brush rather than a comb. However, as time went by, not only was I using a comb, but the hair was becoming limp, lifeless and unmanageable. There was a gradual thinning, rather than a defined balding area, and the hair that I had left was becoming progressively finer. I became obsessed with the problem, and began to look at other people's heads too. I asked myself questions which really could not be explained by the traditional baldness theories.

I was told that the main problems with male pattern baldness were heredity and male hormones. The following facts seemed to me to go against these theories.

1) Studies of women with typical male pattern baldness

show that seventy per cent of such women do not have raised androgen (male hormone) levels.

2) The press tease those with baldness by quoting from various specialists who say that castration may be the only cure for baldness. Where do the women make their androgens, because thirty per cent in the above study *did* have raised androgen levels? Even more to the point, why did these women have a higher level of androgen production?

3) How is it that a strong pattern develops, below which line hair does not normally recede? This can be seen in men with very strong hair growth up to a defined line above which the baldness occurs. If male hormones in the blood stream are the problem, why does their effect end at a certain point, creating such a defined line?

4) Why was it that the drug minoxadil, demonstrated to reverse hair loss in a reasonable percentage of cases, was not a hormone?

5) Countries such as the UK and the USA have one of the highest rates of baldness in the world. What happens to men in these countries to make them lose their hair?

6) The only noticeable change in testosterone levels is during puberty, and from the age of forty-five the level tends to reduce. It follows that baldness should be more predominant in puberty where levels can increase twenty-fold, and slow down as one gets older. The reverse, however, is the case. Why? (See Chapter 1, 'What is Baldness and Why Does It Happen?' for explanations of the current theories, and Chapter 2, 'Andy Bryant's Baldness Theory' for my response to the 'experts'.)

I would sit on commuter trains on the way into work with such questions running through my mind. I noticed that many of my fellow commuters not only suffered baldness, but had dandruff as well. Was there a correlation between dandruff and baldness?

As I began to delve deeper into the subject of testosterone, I found that it operated on a negative feed-back system. If too much testosterone exists in the system then production is slowed down; if too little exists then production is increased. By this mechanism there is a constant level of testosterone always circulating in the system.

I also found to my surprise that women produce about twenty per cent of men's level of the male hormone. This puzzled me, particularly as the castration theory had led me to believe that production would cease after castration. It was also interesting to note that women can convert quite a lot of their male hormone into female hormones, and that their oestrogen neutralizes testosterone.

My research continued, with testosterone taking a back seat while I looked for a common link amongst men with hair and those without, and also amongst women who were losing their hair. I wanted to find out if there was some correlation which did not involve testosterone.

For nearly ten years I studied the way that the mind works, and tried all sorts of mind control techniques to see if they could solve the problem. I looked into areas such as positive thinking, meditation, hypnosis, visualization, Neuro-Linguistic Programming – you name it, I tried it! Still my hair was falling out, and none of these techniques worked.

There was, however, one interesting point: after a very stressful period the hair loss would be more rapid. There would also be a tremendous amount of tension in my neck, my back, my shoulders and in the muscles around my scalp. After the stressful period this tension took some time to disappear. If I was soon again under stress, this tension would effectively be with me on a permanent basis, because I had no time for a recovery period.

I saw numerous television programmes which had people telephoning in speaking to eminent doctors on the subject of baldness. The doctors would explain, in particular to female callers, that it was quite natural for them to lose hair after a stressful event. When questioned about the male hormone they tended to skip over this, focusing on the fact that stress does cause hair loss but that eventually hair lost in this way would grow back.

I found it curious that the doctors did not choose to explain how the raised level of male hormone came about, particularly as medical books indicate that there is a raised level of testosterone production as part of the stress response. Could this be where the raised levels were coming from, as production is not shut down by the same control mechanisms that exist for normal testosterone production?

If a man is under constant stress, his adrenal glands will continually produce testosterone, which would also explain why men who lose hair on their heads also have extra growth of hair on the rest of the body, which testosterone is responsible for. This could also explain why many women who are extremely stressed do suffer an increase in bodily and facial hair.

However, I still kept testosterone at the back of my mind, and would not accept its direct effect on the follicle. Still, I was interested to note that all other research that I had seen and read had been ignoring adrenal production.

The turning point

I was due to have an operation in 1989 to remove a bony growth on one of my toes. I was extremely busy at work (and stressed!) and felt that I could not spare the time to have the operation or to convalesce. But it was getting to the stage where I could hardly walk, as the bone was rubbing against my shoe and causing serious damage to the other toes, so I had to tackle the problem.

During my research on hair loss I went on a weekend course to study hypnosis, so I decided that I would have the operation without an anaesthetic and would control blood loss using hypnosis. My hypnosis teacher was to be present during the operation in case anything went wrong.

The operation was a tremendous success, and I walked out of the hospital an hour later with no pain, no bleeding and no discomfort whatsoever. I thought that if hypnosis could enable me to have an operation by 'turning off' blood and pain, then getting to grips with my hair loss problem should be easy!

I spoke to my hypnotist and others, and tried various techniques to no avail. I was also disappointed to note that some of our successful stage hypnotists were also balding. I was very disappointed that although hypnotists could do some impressive work, they could not solve the problem of baldness. This told me that there must be some very complex physical reason why hair loss occurs. I felt that the answer was to ignore the traditional view of baldness, and to focus on why hypnosis fails.

Within a few weeks of the operation I was off on a ski-ing holiday with a group of friends in France, but I had a nagging thought always in the back of my mind: why was it that a hypnotist can control pain and bleeding, literally switching on or off blood as they choose, but could not reverse baldness?

During the evenings on the holiday my friends and I had various discussions; one of the topics was the 'strange' books I was reading on the plane. I have made it my practice to avoid conversations about religion, politics, hypnosis and cybernetics. The reason is that we all view our lives through the filters of our previous conditioning, created by our upbringing. Our respective points of view on such subjects as hypnosis are largely based on the way we were brought up; our reasoning being based on information that we have been given and stored. The point is that none of us is right or wrong, because we can only base being right or wrong on such conditioning.

One of the books I had been reading on the plane was a remarkable book by Maxwell Maltz, entitled *Psycho-cybernetics*; it caused a lot of interest amongst my friends. I was trying to avoid getting onto the subject because my friends were not into any form of psychology. However, eventually I succumbed, and a friend called Joan and I had a heated discussion on the subject.

Let me explain briefly what cybernetics is. It is partly the study of guided missiles and how they lock on to a given target until they strike. *Psychocybernetics* describes how humans have a servo system, in addition to the conscious mind, which stores these 'targets' – rather like a blueprint for all your beliefs. This servo then drives all your actions on a subconscious level to help you achieve your goals. If you hold a belief firmly enough, your entire body and mind searches continually for an answer and cannot stop until one arrives. The 'guided missile' that goes off track simply uses the data as feed-back to get itself back on track, and it therefore accepts going off track as part of the natural process of finding the target.

People read the negative feed-back as total failure, often giving up just before they've achieved their goal. How, for example, did you learn to ride a bike? The answer is that you learnt to fall off less than you learnt to stay on, and eventually you stayed on most of the time and concluded that you could now ride a bike.

This is a very important principle to understand in connection with hair growth too. As no one had ever grown their hair back before it would be easy to conclude that no one could. If, however, no one had ever ridden a bike you wouldn't try it in the first place. Because you can look at other people riding a bike you too believe that it is possible, and keep trying until you actually succeed.

Joan became rather irritated by our discussion, saying: 'What you're actually telling me is that if you run your mind a certain way, and keep going long enough, you should be able to achieve whatever you set out to.'

I simply replied: 'Yes that is how the theory goes.'

Joan's husband was unmistakably bald, so she simply smiled and said: 'Well, find the cause of baldness – ha ha!'

I replied: 'Yes I'll do that, Joan', and carried on casually talking about the theory.

Joan then interrupted by saying: 'But you have absolutely no medical training. How do you hope to find the answer when some of the finest minds in the world have failed?'

My reply was to say that: 'Using the approach of psycho-cybernetics it doesn't really matter. It will just mean that I will take a little longer to do the background reading to catch up with the doctors. It may even work to my advantage, because I don't have preconceived ideas that in themselves could limit me.'

I was getting frustrated, because Joan really didn't understand the subject, and was looking at it through her own filters. I wanted her at least to understand the filters that *I* was looking through before she continued to challenge me.

This discussion with Joan – and I will always be grateful to her – helped me to decide to make it my goal to discover what causes hair loss, and what could be done to reverse the process. It would not be as simple as merely setting the goal and achieving it; if it *were* that simple, everyone who practises positive thinking would succeed in everything they try to do. The system is more complex, because we have a multitude of goals and targets on a subconscious level, and we have to ensure that a new goal does not conflict with existing ones. For example, I did not enjoy public speaking, yet there would clearly have to be some of that if I were to find the answer to the problem of hair loss. I was very concerned myself about hair loss, and was therefore happy to devote the time and energy necessary to the project. Further, there were many people who would try to discredit me because of my lack of medical training. Was I ready for that?

Having done a sort of mental 'spring clean' to make sure I had no conflicting goals, I resolved that within time I would find the answer – which, indeed, I have done. Along the way I did have to accept, however, that for many men going bald does not present a problem.

I knew that the answer was something so powerful that even a hypnotist could not over-ride it. Testosterone did have some indirect effect, but not in my opinion related to the hair follicle, as I have outlined. I believed that our stress response was a crucial factor, and that testosterone could make a man more aggressive and competitive, thus more likely to use his stress response. There seemed, therefore, to be a number of factors, and not one simple cause.

The contract

The first step in reversing hair loss is for you to agree to devote a given amount of time each day, each week, each month, to re-growing your hair, or else simply close the book for good. You need to decide here and now if re-growing your hair is a priority in your life that will not conflict with your other goals. As you will discover, you are causing your baldness yourself, and will need to spend some time overcoming the problem. You should also determine never to give up until you have a full head of hair.

It will help if you view this as an unbreakable contract with yourself, which you sign and date today.

As with all aspects of life there will be some days when you just cannot manage to do something, so be realistic and accept that 'one day off' is not going to make all your hair fall out again, but at the same time you will need a disciplined approach. There will be many occasions when people will ridicule what you are doing; you may get disheartened, especially if nothing seems to be happening – but you must never give up.

It helps to have some sort of perspective as well, as to how long it will take and what the first signs of hair growth look like. I have given an example in chronological order below.

● Contract signed to re-grow my hair.   01/03/94
● Tension leaving scalp.   14/03/94

- Hair loss begins to slow down.   21/03/94
- Hair appears to have more lift; dandruff   28/03/94
  improving.
- Tension leaving shoulders and back.   01/04/94
- Baby-fine new hair appearing when a small   01/06/94
  torch is shone across scalp. This hair will be
  around the existing hairline.
- More new baby hair, but original baby hair   01/09/94
  maturing, getting longer and darker.
- More new baby hair but original hair get-   01/12/94
  ting longer and darker.
- Quite a noticeable reduction in bald patch.   01/03/95
- A full head of hair.   01/03/96

(Obviously there will be faster and slower growers, depending on the amount of vasoconstriction and scalp tension,
and the effort you put in to reversing the problem.)

Signature

Date

So now that you are re-growing your hair and are never
going to look back, let's have a look at what causes baldness
and how it can be solved.

Chapter 1

What is Baldness and Why Does It Happen?

Types of baldness

There are numerous types of baldness, and each is given a name by the medical profession. I have 'translated' these medical terms into language we can all understand.

1 Alopecia. This simply means baldness.

2 Alopecia Androgenetica. This means that male hormones (androgens) are believed to be causing the baldness. We can simplify this to male hormone baldness.

3 Androgen Dependent Alopecia. A condition as in 2) above, where male hormones are believed to be the cause. Women produce male hormones from their adrenal glands. As many women have a similar baldness pattern to men, they are said to have Androgen (male hormone) Dependent Alopecia (baldness).

4 Diffuse Pattern Alopecia. This is most common in women. The pattern of baldness is more one of thinning hair than balding as such. There is not a defined shiny patch entirely without hair; it is more like every second or third hair were missing, usually across the top of the head and near the front, rarely the sides.

5 Telogen Effluvium. Telogen is the resting stage of hair and rather than shedding up to 90 hairs a day, seven or eight times as much may be lost. Alternatively, the hair may remain in the resting (telogen) stage for a longer period than the usual three months; consequently there is less growing than there should be.

6 Friction Alopecia. This suggests that something has rubbed the hair away, for example a hat worn regularly. The hair is effectively still there but has broken or worn away close to the scalp.

7 Traction Alopecia. Traction means pulling; there are two ways in which this may affect hair growth:

a Some plaited hairstyles pull hard against the follicle, so that the hair is pulled away temporarily or – in more serious cases – the hair follicle becomes permanently damaged.
b The other form can be likened to children who suck their thumbs or have a rag which they use to comfort them. People with this problem subconsciously tug on their hair, and it then falls out. It is habitual behaviour, rather like nailbiting, which people may not realize they are doing.

8 Alopecia Areata. This means baldness in isolated areas. The areas are usually round or oval, and may be there months or years. It is quite common for the hair to grow back again in many cases.

9 Alopecia Totalis. Most or all of the hair on the head is lost.

10 Alopecia Universalis. All or most body hair is lost.

11 Seborrhea. Seborrhea comes from the word sebum, which is the natural oil produced in the sebaceous glands that flows into the hair follicle and up the hair shaft. It means that your scalp is producing too much sebum (oil/grease), and hence you have too oily a scalp. Coupled with the oil is thick dandruff and usually an itchy scalp.

12 Congenital Alopecia. This means baldness from birth.

13 Anagen Effluvium. Anagen is the hair's growing stage; effluvium means that the growing phase has been arrested. Hence the hair has stopped growing. This term is usually used to describe a serious hair-loss problem, where thousands of hairs are lost each day.

14 Deficient Diets. Some forms of baldness may be brought about by poor diet. (See Chapter 3 on diet.)

15 Metabolic Baldness. If the entire metabolism is upset for some reason such as serious illness or sometimes after childbirth, women undergo hormone changes which can cause hair loss. The thyroid gland is the main controller of our metabolism and hence if it is overactive/underactive hair loss can occur.

16 Drug Induced Baldness. Hair loss is a side effect of many drugs, including the contraceptive pill, malaria tablets, drugs used to control thyroidism and acne, hormonal drugs and some antibiotics. The most feared are chemotherapy drugs. Briefly, they are designed to slow down the rapid cellular division of the cancer cells. They travel in the blood, and because hair is made by rapid cellular division, hair loss is very common.

17 Baldness due to Vitamin Excess/Shortage. Excess or shortages of certain vitamins can cause hair loss. (See Chapter 3.)

Current theories on baldness

Traditional views on the main reasons why people go bald can be broken down under the following headings: male hormones, heredity, trauma and age; I outline these views below. I do not accept them, however, as you will see in Chapter 2.

Male hormones

Most of us are aware that men and women have different hormones, which give us our different characteristics. The bulk of the male hormone testosterone is made in the testes, which is evident if they are removed.

In addition to helping testosterone grow pubic hair, underarm hair, hair on faces, ears, nostrils, chins, chests, arms, legs and body, it is believed that Dihydrotestosterone (DHT) shrinks certain target hair follicles in the head. The DHT theory states that, paradoxically, the hormone can increase hair growth on certain parts of the body whilst shrinking it in others. (I do not accept this theory.)

Many experts believe the real culprit is an enzyme called 5 alpha reductace (5AR). It is 5AR which metabolizes testosterone into its derivative DHT.

There are conflicting views on the role of testosterone, however, with some recent scientific papers suggesting that it does not play a significant role in hair loss.

Heredity

As you inherit the colour of your eyes and hair and all other characteristics from your parents, it has been assumed that baldness is hereditary too.

If your father or maternal grandfather is bald, there will be a greater chance that you will become bald too. However, as with all aspects of our inheritance, this is not an absolute certainty, but merely a likelihood.

Clearly we are also likely to inherit our parents' capillary network and the contractile strength of the scalp muscles. In addition our personality types are determined to a large extent by our family background.

It is the inheritance of the stress response and personality type that particularly interest me as far as heredity is concerned. As these are the only two inherited areas that I get people on the programme to adjust, this leads me to believe these are the prime factors in the relationship between heredity and hair loss.

Trauma

A particularly traumatic event may cause hair loss. (Dealing with this form of hair loss is outside the realms of the programme described in the book. Briefly, however, the person affected needs to try to break their accepted association with the painful event, then reframe it so that it causes less stress when they think about it.)

Age

As we all know, men often go bald as they get older. This also happens to women after the menopause; the women's pattern follows the men's, but is more diffuse. (See Chapter 2, p. 28, for *my* reasons why baldness comes about with age.)

In the following chapter I present my response to the 'expert' theories, and also introduce you to what I believe are the real main causes of baldness. Once you can understand and accept *my* theories you will see why the programme for reversing hair loss can work for you.

Chapter 2

Andy Bryant's Baldness Theory

My response to the current theories

I believe that the current theories on why baldness happens
focus too narrowly on factors the 'experts' believe cannot
be changed. These theories do not take into account, the
background and performance of the whole body and therefore fail to see where the real problems lie.

Hormones

Hormones do have an effect, but on the entire body, through
the blood and nervous systems, not just on the hair follicle.
In the study of hair loss the multifactoral evidence about
the differences between men and women is ignored, and
answers concentrate on a small section of activity around
the hair follicle itself. The theory is that testosterone, which
travels in the blood, somehow triggers target hair follicles
to switch off, and at the same time manages to make others
switch on, particularly on the face, chest, legs and arms. I
find this impossible to accept. I believe that the blood

supply has become weaker in the area of traditional male baldness which I refer to from now on as the target zone; hence the fact that the hair still grows, but becomes finer and finer until it eventually appears to have gone completely. I know this to be true, because when I have reversed the process on many people, the hair grows back fine initially and then thicker and stronger as more blood returns to the area.

Let's look at the following information. Studies (see *Brain Sex* in 'Helpful Reading', p. 110) have shown that depending on the levels of testosterone in a developing child, after its first six weeks in the womb the brain grows differently. Men and women are therefore totally different, starting with completely different 'wiring' in the brain. This 'wiring' makes the brain predisposed to act a specific way when a further amount of testosterone is released from puberty onwards.

What we are seeing, therefore, is not testosterone related in isolation to the hair follicle, but its effect on the brain and indeed on the mood of individuals. Injections of testosterone can increase aggressiveness and competitiveness in men, which is the very behaviour that the type 'A' personality exerts and is so damaging to the cardiovascular system (see Chapter 5, 'How to Combat Your Stress', pp. 77–94). The same injections in women do not have such an extreme effect, because their brains are 'wired' differently. So I look at the effect of testosterone on a man's mood, not at its effect on the hair follicle. A man's mood will dictate how he uses his stress response, and hence the degree of scalp tension and vasoconstriction he suffers. These in turn affect the hair growth. The female hormone oestrogen counters the male hormone, but when the level of oestrogen falls during menopause, women develop a similar baldness pattern to men.

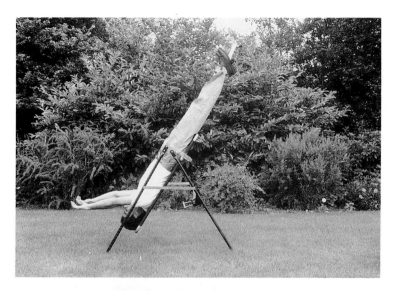

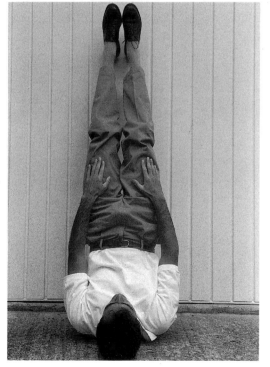

The author
demonstrating how
the inverter works
(*fig 2*)

Promoting blood flow
to the scalp – Exercise
A (*fig 3*)

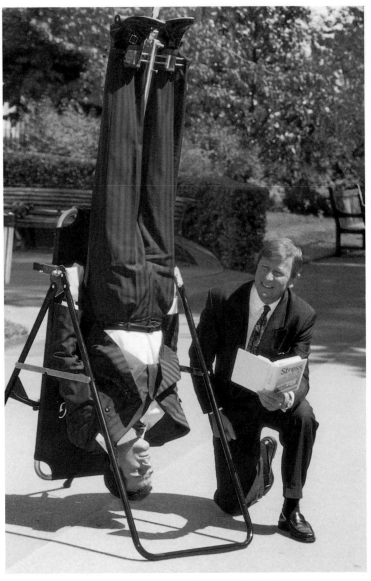

Labour Member of Parliament Bryan Gould, who is currently
undergoing the S.I.D.E.S. course, photographed after the launch of the
Natural Hair Products' programme in May this year (*fig 4*)

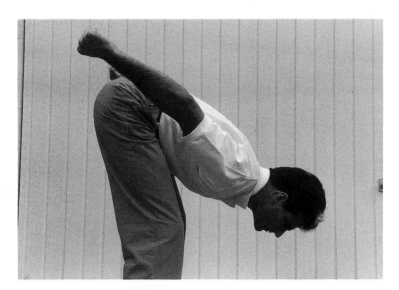

Promoting blood flow to the scalp –
Exercise B (*fig 5*)

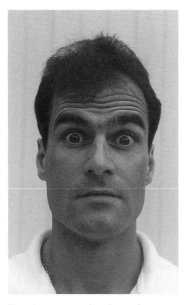

Exercises to control scalp tension –
Exercise C (*fig 7*)

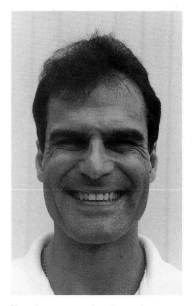

Exercises to control scalp tension –
Exercise D (*fig 8*)

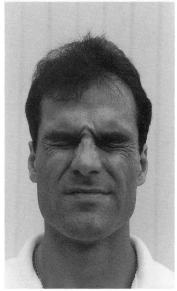

Exercises to control scalp tension –
Exercise E (*fig 9*)

Blood flow and cholesterol

The following table measures the chances of heart attack before age fifty in men and women in the UK.

Age	Male	Female
25	1 in 10	1 in 39
35	1 in 10	1 in 39
45	1 in 11	1 in 40

(DHSS Hospital In-Patients Enquiry 1983)

Why should women have fewer heart attacks? It has been believed that cholesterol plays a major role, but I was interested to read the work of Meyer Friedman and Ray Roseman in *Type A Behaviour and Your Heart.* They conclude that chronic excess discharge and circulation of catecholamines (adrenalin and noreadrenalin) may be the chief factor in the decay of the arteries and thrombosis.

On the cholesterol question, Friedman and Roseman conclude that they had seen coronary heart disease erupt in many people whose blood insulin levels and metabolism of cholesterol, fat and sugar were quite normal. But rarely had they witnessed the onset of heart disease in a person who did not know or suspect that their rate of manufacture and secretion of catecholamines had been increased.

I do not wish to be misunderstood on this point: I am *not* saying that the cholesterol issue should be ignored, but that the priorities are: 1 Keeping down levels of adrenalin and noradrenalin; 2 keeping cholesterol levels down. (It is worth noting that ninety per cent of cholesterol is manufactured by the liver, so ten per cent comes via diet. I am interested in controlling the liver's production via the stress response, and then paying attention to diet.)

A deeper look at cholesterol

The cholesterol issue is a controversial one as outlined above. The real problem area is arteriosclerosis. This begins with injuries to the lining of the arteries; whilst the cause has not been proven conclusively, the following are known to be contributory factors: cigarette smoking; high blood pressure; and high cholesterol levels.

These are within your control, in that you can give up smoking; controlling your adrenalin will aid blood pressure and cholesterol levels.

Too great a level of cholesterol in the blood will result in fatty deposits in the arteries, and a loss of elasticity in the artery walls, thus eventually hindering blood flow.

Imagine cholesterol being like candle wax when it arrives in the blood. The body cannot absorb it in that form, so the liver 'coats' it in a protein. There are known to be more than a dozen such proteins; one is Low Density Lipoprotein (LDL), which is thought to collect the cholesterol and deposit it in the cells. Another is High Density Lipoprotein (HDL), which is thought to help the body eliminate it. It is logical to conclude that women, who statistically have fewer heart attacks, should have more HDLs, and are producing fewer catecholamines by having a different stress response from that of men. Similarly, genetically men could be 'wired' to have more LDLs or less HDLs. Clearly, your stress response will raise your cholesterol level.

In this context it is interesting to note that breast milk has more fat and milk sugar and less protein than cow's milk. Whilst an infant's liver cannot readily absorb the fats and calcium in cow's milk, it can absorb nearly ninety-eight per cent of the fat in mother's milk. In adults this cholesterol might be harmful; in an infant it appears to promote the secretion of enzymes that keep blood cholesterol levels down. In the early months of development, a high cholesterol requirement is paramount for the baby's rapidly developing nervous system. A logical conclusion is that if a woman has to manufacture milk that is so high in cholesterol and fat, and at the same time ensure the baby secretes the enzymes that 'park' the cholesterol in the cells rather than allow it to clog up the baby's blood, her own body will take on some of those characteristics. It also explains how after menopause she follows the male pattern of heart complaint and baldness.

(The focus of the programme is to increase blood circulation to the finest capillaries in the scalp. Clearly, anything that restricts the flow inside the arteries and capillaries, as in the case of arteriosclerosis, will reduce the blood flow.)

Heredity

Rather than as described in Chapter 1, I believe that the blueprint of the *whole* body may lean towards baldness, taking in our blood flow, neurology and even psychological factors such as temperament.

From a young age we are continually mimicking those around us. This can be seen in how quickly children copy the responses or gestures of their parents – or indeed suppress particular responses because of a parent. Having formed a set of beliefs at a young age, these beliefs are very rarely upgraded or questioned. For example, if you become stressed over little things, why not change this? Are you a workaholic? Could you earn as much money doing less in a more organized and relaxed way? Were your parents type 'A' personalities? (See Chapter 5 for details on type 'A' personalities.)

Psychology has taught us that dramatic changes in personality can be brought about by trauma, fear or misinterpretation. These features cannot be ignored in the baldness equation. Whilst not strictly hereditary, a pattern of psychological behaviour is passed down from generation to generation. I am interested in how we manage our learned stress response as outlined earlier; I believe that this is the single most important factor underlying baldness.

Age

I believe baldness comes about with age due to a gradual clogging up of the capillary network; eventually blood and lymph flow to the capillaries in part of the scalp ceases altogether. The following table shows how average blood pressure readings increase with age. If a 'pipe' narrows, greater pressure is needed to drive the fluid through it. Similarly, if the arterial walls begin to fur up, like the inside of a kettle, they become less elastic. Briefly, the larger arteries expand and then recoil, driving blood into the small arteries; these in turn expand and recoil. When the elasticity is lost, the flow is more difficult, requiring more pumping action.

Mean systolic pressure
(with standard deviations rounded)

Age	Men	Women
20–24	110–137	104–129
40–44	114–144	110–144
60–64	119–167	122–166
80–84	119–171	133–185

Rather than accepting that baldness or thinning hair inevitably comes about with age you *can* do something about it.

The causes of baldness

In order to work successfully through the hair loss reversal and restoration programme it is important for you to understand just why I believe baldness comes about. Then you will see the basis for each aspect of the programme as a whole.

I have been able to identify three prime causes of baldness:

1 Blood has difficulty getting through to the hair follicle owing to vasoconstriction and muscular tension.
2 The blood that does get through carries with it insufficient nutrients for hair growth.
3 The waste products from cellular activity find it difficult to drain away from the scalp through the lymphatic system.

In themselves these appear to be very simple problems to overcome, so why has it taken so long for anyone to find the answer? The reason is that baldness is a progressive condition that we allow our bodies to get into; it can be reversed, but like whole nations bent on a course of action it is difficult, once embarked on it, to get off the conveyer belt. Only when you have been able to step off the conveyer belt and examine the situation from an independent point of view, do the answers look obvious.

Baldness is not a separate condition, but an external sign of the condition of the body as a whole. When I have spoken to specialists on the subject they point out that if you cut the head it will bleed. If there were insufficient blood then this would not happen, they believe. The specialist does this from his position on the conveyer belt, missing the point of what is being said. He views the world through his own filters of training and environment, and finds it difficult to open his mind to new possibilities.

In my early days of overcoming baldness many doctors put forward this 'cut and bleed theory' to me. I got so frustrated at one point that I asked a doctor whether he would like a demonstration of the fact that the body does not bleed when it chooses not to, wherever you cut it. He agreed, so I arranged that he should put a pin in whatever part of his body he chose and see that he would not bleed. Having successfully demonstrated this point it changed his entire view of how the body operates; he could then begin to open his mind to what I was saying.

For you it must be the same: open your mind to new possibilities, do not judge anything I say until you have experimented with it yourself. If you hold in front of you your existing ideas like filters you will not learn anything new from this book, but simply have reflected back to you your own ideas and views.

Vasoconstriction

Vasoconstriction is where the body closes down the finer capillaries, to divert blood to other areas of the body. Let us follow the journey of a few blood cells from the heart through the body into the hair follicle. The route passes through the heart, through the aorta, up either the left or right common carotid artery, through the external artery, branching into the superior temporal artery; after that medical textbooks become a little vague. The reason for this is that the blood capillaries branch off into literally hundreds then thousands of smaller capillaries, until eventually the hundred thousand or so hairs on the average head have their own little blood supply.

It is the finer vessels at the end of the journey that do not allow blood to flow through them, not the larger vessels – which explains the cut and bleed theory. The blood flow gets restricted in the smaller capillaries for two reasons.

1 The body has chosen to close the smaller vessels and move the blood to areas that at the time it considered to be more important. This is known as vasoconstriction, where the smaller capillaries are restricted by muscles within them that close them tight. The body can choose any small area it wishes and shut the blood flow down, taking the blood instead to areas of higher priority.
2 The muscle tension in the muscles that pull down on the scalp is greater than the pressure inside the blood vessels, therefore cutting off the flow of blood.

If you can learn how to control these two elements, letting

the blood flow into the capillaries again, your hair will begin to grow. Learning this lesson is very difficult, however, because it means adjusting how we automatically conduct our lives. The muscle tension and blood movements are fired off subconsciously; learning how to override these subconscious commands is not easy, particularly as they are driven by the fight or flight mechanism, which controls our physical responses.

My approach is to use a system which jump-starts or over-rides the subconscious, while you are learning to control blood flow and muscle tension.

As I have said above, depending on the perceived requirements of different parts of the body, blood will be diverted from one area to another for as long as the brain considers it necessary. Brains take priority in the body's pecking order, so brains will always direct flow to themselves first. Lower on the priority list is the hair, taking its place in the order way behind areas such as the heart, lungs, kidneys, liver and spleen. It follows that if we have a defined amount of blood within our system when smaller capillaries are closed the pressure will increase in other areas of the body.

Fight or flight

In evolutionary terms it was not so long ago that we all lived in a world of real physical danger, having literally to fight for our lives. When faced with danger it is 'all hands on deck' for battle stations, so that we may survive. The fuel required for fighting needs to go to the major muscle groups of the arms, the legs, the shoulders, the back, the jaw, the chest, the heart and the lungs. The fuel is blood sugar and oxygen. Emergency supplies are taken from the liver, and all work shut down temporarily in areas of lower importance. The blood flow is therefore diminished in the digestive tract and the skin and hair, and the heart increases its pace, causing the lungs to draw in more oxygen.

Design fault in modern man

In our modern, fast-living society the bulk of what disturbs us and provokes this response is not physical but psychological. The problem with our alerting system is that it does not recognize the difference between a physical or emotional stress, and undergoes the same changes whatever the cause. Today we are living lives which are ever more stressful, and many people run their bodies constantly at this super-charged, battle-station mode.

In doing so we affect our hair in the following ways:

1 The blood supply that has been shut down never gets a chance to return because of continual stresses; therefore the hair is not properly nourished.

2 The blood is thicker and travels at a slower pace, finding it more difficult to enter the smaller capillaries once they do open again.

3 I believe that clotting factors released in this thicker blood cause clotting in the capillaries in the target zone. This is caused by the fact that the thicker blood, holding more clotting agents, is held tightly in one area for a prolonged period by high muscular tension.

4 The smooth muscles inside the capillaries need fuel (ATP) and oxygen to drive them (see pp. 40–41). Unlike skeletal muscles smooth muscles cannot work without oxygen, and do not store a supply of fuel. They are able to lock closed and stay closed when the fuel reserve runs out. It follows that a capillary which is in competition with a muscle that has vasodilated (opened) its capillaries is not going to be able to open until it gets its fuel.

5 Cholesterol furs up the arteries. Blood flow is usually aided by elastic recoil in the artery walls. If this elasticity is lost owing to the furring up of the arteries it is more difficult for blood to flow. Greater pressure is therefore needed to drive the blood around the system at all times, which taxes the system as a whole.

6 Muscular tension pulling across the target zone stops the blood flow from entering and feeding the follicle.

7 The digestive tract has been tampered with, so that correct nutrients are not supplied on a regular basis.

8 We burn up our vital vitamin and mineral reserves during our battle-stations mode, so that the hair is starved. Much damage has been caused by the system during battle stations and therefore when the system should return to normal a lot of repair work has to be done in the major organs before our hair will receive its quota of nutrients and vitamins.

Inverting the body for optimum blood flow

The way that I have achieved such dramatic hair growth is to put optimum blood flow back into the scalp; this is done by totally inverting the body, with the aid of an inversion device (see Figure 2 in plate section). The way the device is designed, anyone using it is totally in control of the level of inversion; this is because of the machine's fine balance, and the angle altering as you raise your arms above the centre of gravity. If you were not in control in this way the body could become distressed, which would bring about a restriction in blood flow.

There are receptors in the neck and chest which measure slight changes in blood pressure and open the peripheral capillaries to reduce the pressure if it becomes too high. I have therefore chosen a design which gradually increases the pressure; some days the body will need less pressure than others to cause this vasodilation. Not only is it easier for the blood to run downhill towards the capillaries, but they are opened still further by the receptors trying to drop the pressure elsewhere in the system. Initially an angle of forty-five degrees will suffice. Week by week the angle is fractionally altered so that the pressure continually builds, assuring you of a consistent vasodilation.

I recommend that you invert every morning and evening, with the following schedule.

	Inversion time (seconds)	Position (degrees)
Week 1	25	45
Week 2	30	65
Week 3	30	75
Week 4	30	90

Once you have reached the ninety-degree angle, gradually increase your inversion time, to a total of three minutes. Remember, the capillaries in your head have probably never had this pressure exerted on them. *Do not* speed up inversion time from thirty seconds to three minutes. Your body will tell you when you have had enough! It is not a race or challenge, where you have to reach three minutes as fast as possible. (See p. 111 for information on how to purchase the correct type of inverter.)

Safety and the inverter

If you have, or have ever had, any of the following conditions or are in any doubt whatsoever, it is advisable to consult your medical practitioner before commencing the Hair Growth Programme.

- Causes of back pain that are not the common ones, e.g., cancer and tuberculosis
- Damaged or loose ankle and knee joints
- Hypertension (high blood pressure)
- Brittle bone disease
- Unhealed fractures
- Artificial hip joints or lower limb prostheses
- History of heart attack or angina
- Cerebral thrombosis (stroke)
- Retinal detachment
- Glaucoma
- Hiatus hernia
- Osteoporosis
- Aneurysm
- Pregnancy
- Obesity
- Diabetes
- Vertigo

If you cannot afford an inverter

The price of the specially designed inverter (around £300 at the time of going to press) may not be within everyone's reach, although for optimum hair growth a full, controlled inversion is desirable. However, the following posture will give you some blood flow to the scalp until you are able to purchase a suitable inverter.

Exercise A If you put your legs and arms up against the wall as shown in Figure 3 this will help the blood flow.

Exercise B If you bend your head down towards your toes and raise your arms behind you as in Figure 5, this will also create increased blood flow.

The right shampoo

The shampoo that I use has three important tasks:

1 To be as near as possible to the pH balance of the scalp itself, i.e., 5.0–5.6.
2 To clean the hair and scalp with a natural disinfectant. The shampoo thus kills bacteria and fungal infections.
3 To increase the blood circulation in the scalp.

Make sure you use a shampoo that has the above functions. (See p. 111 for details of how to contact the NHP, as you can buy the recommended shampoos by mail order.)

Summary

During a stressful period our bodies respond by diverting the blood away from the hair follicle to areas that they consider more appropriate. If we use our stress response too often, the blood travelling around the body is thicker than it should be; the body is also slightly dehydrated, and has a raised cholesterol level. Eventually permanent damage is done, so that no blood gets through to the follicle even when we are not in a 'vasoconstriction mode'. Through the programme, therefore, we are increasing the pressure slowly, opening the capillaries and forcing blood back into the damaged area.

The muscles

To understand the next section, on muscular tension, you need to know something about the body's muscle systems. The muscles of the body can be divided into two types: skeletal and smooth muscles.

Skeletal muscles

Skeletal muscles resemble electric cable in their structure. On the outside there is a connective tissue wrapping, like the insulation of a cable. Inside run strands of muscle fascicles which have their own outer layer of connective tissue wrapping. These resemble the wires inside a cable. Inside the muscle fascicles are thinner muscle fibres (muscle cells) with their own outer coating, like thinner wires.

Finally, the muscle cells contain myofibrils, which in turn contain myofilaments that cause muscular contraction. This is like the fine wire of an electric plug, with the myofilaments representing the tiny copper strands inside the thin wires. Here the analogy ends, because the myofilaments are very complex in structure, and create the contractile strength of the muscle.

The individual wires are units in their own right, with their own blood supply and lymphatic system. They are anchored together at varying points so that movement within creates a movement of the entire muscle.

It is inside the myofilaments that men and women differ so dramatically. In sport, men can run faster, swim faster and lift greater weights, although women have the same muscle groups. The difference is due to the contractile force of the muscles (so complex so as to be beyond the scope of this book).

In simple terms, two different proteins make up the myofilaments. The thinnest are made of a protein called actin, and the thick ones mainly of a protein called myosin. These thin and thick myofilaments do not run continuously, but overlap and slide past one another. Chemical reactions cause heads on the thick filaments to attach to the thin ones, pulling themselves along. It is not unlike velcro, in that hundreds of these heads grip on the thin filaments, move along and then more heads attach as the ones behind them break free and move along further.

Male hormones cause men simply to have more thick filaments and more red blood cells to oxygenate them; hence in men there are more thick filaments pulling at the same time.

The fuel for contraction is Adenoisine Triphosphate (ATP) which is the same fuel used by all cells for their energy. Unlike other cells, muscles break down the ATP into a finer compound; this releases a high energy compound, which bonds the phosphate molecules. A muscle can run on different fuels: in its resting stage it runs on a breakdown of fatty acids; when a muscle is exercised it adds oxygen to its fuel. It is, however, possible for a muscle to work without oxygen for a period of time which it does by burning nearly twenty times more fuel.

It is for this reason that a muscle stores so much fuel in the form of glycogen. Without sufficient oxygen, glycogen converts to lactic acid, causing that pain in the calf muscles experienced when one first goes on a long distance run, for example. Lactic acid in the body signals the body to take up more oxygen. The term for the usual oxygenated fuel is aerobic; unoxygenated fuel is called anaerobic.

Smooth muscles

Smooth muscles exist in the digestive tract, walls of arteries, veins and the lymphatic system for example. They have more thick filaments, making strong contraction possible. Smooth muscles cannot operate anaerobically, and need a continual flow of oxygen. However, when depleted of ATP they effectively lock their 'velcro grips' until ATP is supplied again and the grips can be broken. In this way, without utilizing too much energy, the muscles can hold a strong contraction for long periods of time.

It is interesting to note a dilemma which exists in our target zone. Assume a capillary is closed in a stressful period by vasodilation, and simply locks out owing to a lack of ATP. The skeletal muscles in the scalp and neck are in spasm, having been firing continually for weeks or months. The tension created stops the blood flow to the scalp and hence the flow of ATP; the locks stay in place, restricting further blood flow through the capillaries.

Muscular tension

To understand what causes tension in the scalp you also need to have a brief understanding of the face and head muscles and how they operate. Interestingly, the areas that have muscle (section A on figure 6) rarely go bald, and the area of the head without muscle (section B) is the area

that does go bald. If you completely shade in all of section
A on the line drawing, the traditional male pattern baldness
becomes obvious.

What you will find at times of rapid hair loss is that the
scalp will be tight. The muscles that surround the scalp all
pull downwards, creating pressure across the sheet of ten-
don covering the scalp. After a prolonged period, the
muscles lock into spasm and stay locked, so that a tight
scalp becomes permanent. This tension also spreads to the
neck and between the shoulders.

When our bodies undergo stress, or to be more precise,
when they view what is happening around them as stressful,
they immediately go into battle stations ready to fight or
run away. To give a simple example, you awake in the

MALE PATTERN BALDNESS (Figure 6)

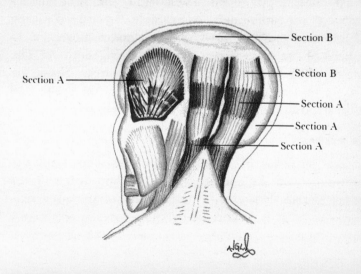

middle of the night and walk in the dark to the toilet. You spot a shadow in the hallway which you are certain is an intruder; your heart begins to pound, and your breathing races. The intruder does not move; your senses tune themselves up, listening for the slightest sound and looking for a clearer picture in the dark. You then remember that you left your coat hanging in that position in the hallway! Whilst the panic is over externally, internally it will take your body some time to recover because of the cocktail that has been released into the blood stream, and the muscular tension created, gearing it up for action.

In such a situation it was not what was happening to you, but how you presented the information to yourself that caused the body to go into full alert. This response is subconscious, and at its peak the scalp, back and neck muscles automatically tense for action.

A vital step in re-growing your hair is to break the muscular tension in the scalp. You can do this by following the exercises on pp. 46–48. These cause groups of muscles to move at the same time. For example, if you keep raising and lowering your eyebrows, you will notice movement in the back of the scalp if you place your fingers there. The muscles which are used to raise the eyebrows share the same nerve with the muscle at the back of the scalp, and pull in opposite directions, thus creating tension.

The nerves

For the purposes of understanding this book and the programme you do not need in-depth knowledge of the nervous system. However, to understand what causes muscular tension, it is important to know something about a rather antiquated part of the system called fusimotor nerves.

In our primeval state, part of our stress response was to signal certain nerves to put muscles into tension ready for action. As we evolved, we transferred much muscular activity to the central control of the brain, which overrides the fusimotor system. Take writing as an example. As a child you had little coordination, as you had not practised using the muscles necessary to write. If anything, you used too much muscular effort, and only gradually learned to inhibit certain muscles as you refined control of others. As an adult, most of the time you do not even think about writing; the muscles have been so well trained that the bulk of their control has been transferred directly to the subconscious. So it is with most things: we are clumsy to start with, and then gradually refine our movements.

Most of our muscles have been trained in this manner, so that the fusimotor system rarely has too much influence over these finely tuned muscles. However, the muscles of our back, neck and scalp are not so finely tuned, and do tense up when we use our primeval alerting system (the stress response).

Breaking the tension

There are three levels you will have to go through to banish this tension for good.

1 Short term you can distort the muscles (as described later): this will quieten down the nervous activity.
2 Exercises which stretch the muscles, causing them to fire off different nerves which in turn quieten them down, are to be done daily. In addition, you will need to do some

relaxation exercises, which will calm the muscles and signal to the body that you are not under stress.

3 You are only firing these muscles as a stress response, and are therefore going to have to spend some considerable time dealing with the areas of stress in your life and the way you automatically respond to them. (This in turn will stop the muscles firing off in the first place.)

Initially you should do the stretching and relaxation exercises daily. After a while you may find that the tension has left you, and only returns when there is a stressful problem on hand. It follows that if you can learn to control your stress eventually you can stop doing the exercises on a daily basis, using them only at difficult times. The object of the exercises is to put an end to the vicious circle of muscle tension and spasm producing pain and a reduced blood flow to the target zone. In addition this will free the lymphatic system to do its job of draining away waste products effectively (see pp. 53–55).

Painful areas

Certain areas in the body are painful when touched; this pain may vary from light discomfort to being totally unbearable. What happens is that as a muscle moves into spasm there is a lack of blood and oxygen feeding it; it then produces waste products, which in turn send out pain signals. Thereafter follows a cycle of more muscular tension, more pain, more waste products and more pain signals.

There is much controversy over what these painful areas are. I simply know that they are there and do not worry too much why! My own hypothesis is that they are areas in the muscle that do not shut down after a lot of fusimotor

activity. If you treat that as the cause, and send the
appropriate message back to the nervous system to have
them 'switched off', you can guess that you are close to the
truth when they switch off every time. As the object of the
exercise is to switch them off, I will focus on that and not
actually what they are.

If you place your fingers in the temple regions, and open
and close your jaw, you will find the muscle there that is
linked to jaw movement. Press along the length of the
muscle – you may find an area that is quite painful. The
pain will increase at the centre of the muscle. Place your
strongest finger, or thumb, in the most painful area; gradually increase the pressure until the pain is as much as you
can stand. After holding that pressure for three minutes, the
pain will slowly subside. What is happening is that you are
distorting the centre of the muscle, therefore causing the
fusimotor nerves to give different signals to the brain,
shutting down the nervous activity. If the pain is not caused
by fusimotor activity, but is referred pain due to damaged
joints, or a trapped nerve or stress which is permanent, the
pain will gradually return until the cause is dealt with.
However, the scalp and neck exercises on pp. 46–50 will
control it. Having removed the pain it is logical to control
the stress and therefore stop the fusimotor activity from
over-burdening the system.

Exercises to control scalp tension

The exercise routine that follows should be carried out on
a daily basis for the first three months. Even if you believe
that you have broken the scalp tension, it is a good idea to
keep doing the exercises. By doing so you will strengthen

the muscles themselves, thereby promoting greater blood flow to the region. **N.B.** If you find that any of these exercises cause you any pain or discomfort, stop doing them immediately; if the pain persists consult your GP showing him or her exactly what you have been doing on the programme.

Scalp muscle exercises

Sit comfortably in a chair, or lie on the floor or on a bed, and close your eyes. Take ten slow deep abdominal breaths to quieten your system down and oxygenate your blood. By an abdominal breath I mean raise the abdomen as you breathe in and suck the abdomen up and in as you breathe out. It sometimes helps if you place one hand on your abdomen and the other hand on your chest so that you can ensure that only the abdomen moves, and not the chest. Inhale for the count of five in your mind and then hold the breath in, extending the abdomen for the count of twenty, and then exhale to the count of ten. Between each exercise do one abdominal breath in this way.

Exercise C (Figure 7) Raise the eyebrows as high as you can; this will cause deep furrows in the brow. Hold for the count of eight then give one last push up with the eyebrows and relax.

Exercise D (Figure 8) Put your hands over your ears and feel the fleshiness of the muscles over the ears as you do the following exercise. Open your mouth in an artificially wide toothy grin; raise the cheek muscles at the same time as high as you can, and close your eyes tightly. This should create some movement in the muscles over the ears. Hold for the count of eight, and then exert just a little more pressure before relaxing.

Exercise E (Figure 9) Pull the eyebrows down, screwing up the nose and closing the eyes as you do so. Remember to hold the position for a count of eight and then give a last little pull on the muscles before you relax.

Try placing your fingers in the traditional receding hairline area above your brow as you do this exercise and Exercise C; you will feel the muscles in that region contract and relax. It is these frontal muscles that cause the tension over the receding hairline area in conjunction with the muscles over the ears. The joint tension created by the opposing pulls of these two muscles brings about the pressure necessary to stem the blood flow, gradually causing the hairline to recede.

One side of your hairline may be receding further than the other side, and if so there will be a corresponding differential in tension in the left and right side of your head.

Exercise F Open your mouth quite wide and move it from side to side as far as it will comfortably go. Then move it backwards and forwards, so that your lower teeth protrude further than the top teeth.

Exercise G Bite gently with your back teeth a couple of times.

Carry out a further ten deep slow abdominal breaths, breathing in for five, holding for twenty, and breathing out for ten before proceeding to the neck exercises. The object of the combination of the exercises and relaxed breathing is that it calms the whole system down.

Neck exercises

The following exercises must be carried out sitting on a chair, preferably with a low back, or a stool.

When I first show people the neck exercises that follow, they look at me as if to say: 'How can such simple little movements do all the good you are claiming?' The simple answer is that I do not claim anything for the exercises, I just report what benefits my clients have received. Try the exercises for yourself to see how you too can benefit.

It may help if I explain something about the way the neck and back work. The spine is an alternating series of discs and vertebrae, surrounded by a mass of nerves, with the spinal chord at its centre. Throughout most of the day gravity pushes down on our bodies, causing outward pressure on the discs in your spine. A disc is comprised predominantly of water; living in this water are specialized living cells. These cells require food and oxygen; in addition they produce waste products that need to be passed out of the system.

Discs do not have their own blood supply within them, because the pressure inside the disc may be greater than that in the blood supply. If the pressure falls in the disc, fluid is sucked in, and if it is too great, fluid seeps out. The best position for sucking fluid into the disc is when you are lying flat on the floor, and the worst position for pushing fluid out of the disc is when you are leaning forward (typing, for example). When you stand upright fluid is neither being sucked into nor being squeezed out of the disc. However, a further mechanism also helps. This system is called diffusion. It is where a chemical solution spreads from an area of high concentration to an area of low concentration. By this process nutrients are taken through the disc itself, and the waste products from the internal activity are passed out through the disc wall.

The best aid to diffusion is movement; the neck exercises regenerate the living force inside the cell itself. This keeps the vertebrae well clear of the nerves, which if trapped aggravate muscular tension.

Exercise H Starting with the head in an upright central position, tilt your head as far forward as it will comfortably go; hold for a count of six. *Gently* tip your head backwards slightly, and hold for a count of six. Now tip your head forward again, but this time move it slightly to the right as you extend it forward; hold for the count of six and then move back to the centre position. From the centre position tip your head backwards again slightly, for a count of six, and then forward, this time taking it fractionally to the right.

You may experience a cracking and crunching sound during this or the other neck exercises; this should not concern you greatly (unless painful, in which case consult your GP), and will subside after a couple of weeks.

Exercise I With your eyes looking forward, tip your head to the left so that the left ear travels down towards the shoulder. Hold for the count of six and then return to the centre.

Exercise J From the centre position repeat Exercise I to the right hand side.

Exercise K From the centre position turn your head to the left as far as it will comfortably go, as if you were looking over your left shoulder; hold for a count of six. Then return to the centre position.

Exercise L Repeat Exercise K to the right.

Many people believe that the other parts of the programme are the most important, and tend to skip over this area. However, the discipline you employ in the early days on these exercises has a profound effect on the overall speed of your success. As with any form of exercise, you should remember that the muscles have not been worked for a long time, and you should never overwork them. Gradually, over a period of three months, build up to three repetitions of each exercise twice a day.

The tension in your scalp should be monitored regularly. You will find that it quickly diminishes as you carry out these exercises, *morning* and *evening* without fail.

Massage

You have seen that blood flow clearly has an important role in scalp health, as does lymphatic drainage. So massage theoretically should be of assistance. I spent a whole year having a regular back and neck massage every week to no avail. The tension in my back was such that painful lumps would appear together with knotty muscle fibre. Whilst the masseur could break the tension within an hour the tension would return within a few days. Having got to the root cause and begun to deal with it, I now have no such problem, and enjoy a massage from time to time without discomfort.

I do recommend that you reward yourself from time to time with massage, concentrating on the back, neck and scalp muscles.

You can gently massage the scalp muscles with the pads of your fingers. Once the scalp begins to loosen, run your fingers through your hair over the muscles and grip the hair between the fingers and palms as near to the scalp as possible – that is, as close to the base of the hair as possible. Now move the scalp gently back and forth and up and down. The muscles will quickly loosen with repeated movement.

As discussed earlier, there are no muscles in the target zone so there is little point massaging it too much. Light squeezing with the pads of the fingers so that the scalp is being pulled upwards as if off the head will suffice.

A very quick way to break tension in the scalp is to 'fire' the muscles of the scalp as outlined earlier in the chapter. The tension is held in the muscle only for a fraction of a second. It helps to place the pads of the fingers high on the traditional receding hairline area as you fire the muscles. It feels as if you are doing the reverse of a massage, in that the fingers move around as muscular contraction pulls them in different directions.

Do not, however, overdo this exercise. Twenty to thirty seconds is long enough: blood flow should be to the scalp, not the muscles.

Insufficient nutrients in the blood

A hair is comprised mainly of amino acids (protein); hence we need to include protein in our diets on a daily basis. We need no more than 2oz daily, so we also need to look at what other constituents are needed in our diet. (See Chapter 3, 'Your Eating Habits', for an in-depth look at food and drink in the programme.)

I am sure that by now you will see that the different aspects of the programme are linked. Restoring blood flow to the scalp is essential, but giving that blood the best possible constituents is also important.

The aim of the programme is simultaneously to increase the blood supply (in an artificial way) to promote hair growth, whilst dealing with the true cause of constriction. The blood flow will be returned naturally to the target zone for a maximum amount of time each day; eventually we move away from an artificial way of jump-starting the blood flow back to the area. The advantage with this approach is that even if you are not very good at controlling the constriction your hair will still grow. This reward may be enough to encourage you to try a little harder! In short, the methods I use to jump-start the hair growth are powerful enough to over-ride the constriction in the short term.

It is logical to conclude that if the nutrients that are needed to provide healthy heads of hair are increased permanently, then you will have sufficient in the blood at the time you jump-start the system to obtain growth.

For you to understand this, let me explain another concept. The brain is always aware of where it is deficient in a substance, and exactly what nutrients are coming into the body. Imagine the brain labelling all the tiny particles that it breaks the food into, posting them to areas of greatest need. Inevitably, it would look after itself and the vital organs such as the heart, liver, kidneys and lungs long before the hair. It follows that if the body is regularly stressed, as previously discussed, with the blood consequently being diverted to areas considered more important for survival, even if the hair was next on the list for nutrients it will miss its position in the queue. By the time the blood flow returns to the hair follicle, so much damage may have been caused by the body's constant state of alertness that the hair remains at the bottom of the brain's priorities for nutrients. (See Chapter 3, 'Your Eating Habits', pp. 61–62 for helpful information on nutrient deficiency and sources.)

Lymphatic drainage

Blood travels around the body in a closed system of blood vessels. The capillary walls are semi-permeable (leaky); fluid similar to blood plasma seeps through the capillary walls and circulates throughout the tissues to take food, oxygen and water to the living cells. Waste products from the cellular activity are taken in this fluid into the veins or the lymphatic system. The veins have a pump, the heart, driving the blood around the system; lymph has no such pump, and is drained away via lymphatic vessels. The smallest lymph vessels arise in the tissues as blind tubes which, like a stream, form a network running into larger and larger vessels. The fluid in these vessels is known as lymph which flows through the body in a one-way system driven by either gravitational pull or muscular activity. The muscles create pressure on the outside walls of the vessel, which drives the fluid around inside; valves stop it flowing backwards. Thus as long as there is muscular activity there is one-way movement of fluid along the vessels. It follows that if the scalp is held tightly in tension there is a restricted flow in the lymphatic system, with a consequent build-up of toxins.

On all the balding heads that I have examined, there has always been complete atrophy of the scalp in the balding area. The scalp gradually compresses until it feels almost woody. When you begin to reverse the balding process, the scalp regenerates and becomes fleshy once again. This does not happen overnight, and will take many months.

The nerves that fire the muscles in the head and jaw also control the face. This atrophy can be seen in facial muscles which become locked in spasm, showing for example in a deep furrowed brow or in harsh lines underneath the eyes.

Those who have followed the programme for a year or more have found that there is a defined softening in these facial muscles as the spasms are released and muscles regain their mobility. The soft contours of the muscles return and stronger muscles develop. There is sometimes a considerable improvement in facial appearance as a result; a reversal of ageing appears to take place also, with an overall improvement in complexion.

Improvements in the complexion happen so often in the early months that many men on the programme found that their partners were joining in just for this benefit. It is worth passing *The Baldness Cure* on to your partner for the dual purpose of improving her complexion and reducing muscular tension. Women do suffer from male pattern baldness, but are offered some protection by their hormones until after the menopause. If your spouse simply follows the programme just for her complexion, when she passes the menopause she should not suffer baldness.

There are no specific exercises to aid the lymphatic system: the programme itself aids lymphatic drainage when you work on muscle tension and improve blood flow.

Summary

To recap, baldness occurs not through heredity, nor as a result of the effect of testosterone on the hair follicles in the target zone. Rather it is caused because of: poor blood flow to the scalp (from a number of causes); insufficient nutrients in the blood; poor drainage of waste products through the lymphatic systems. These are problems that can be solved, as you have already seen, by following the hair growth programme.

Chapter 3

Your Eating Habits

Let's not use the word diet, because it is associated with pain and suffering. On the other hand, we all have eating habits, and the way we habitually eat is what I am interested in. My experience is that when you go on a diet, the very fact that you *have* to change habitual patterns, which are often difficult to do for social reasons, makes us fail. Our bodies may read the common famine/feast approach to a diet as a message to store as much of our food as possible for the next famine (diet) period. This means we can eat less and actually gain weight – that's why so many people give up.

I think you should change your eating habits by eating more. Sounds like a good idea: let's eat more and lose weight! That is not what the change of eating habits is intended to do, but it is a side benefit many of those following the programme have reported. They even lose weight in all the 'right' places.

Let me explain what I am trying to do:

1 The building blocks that your body needs for repair work on your scalp can be obtained from a high water-content diet, plus a *small* amount of protein. These building blocks are carried in our blood, which is water-based.

2 The water content of the diet will aid the drainage of waste products through the lymphatic system; lymph is also water-based. This will help the body to function more healthily, and deliver nutrients to the hair follicles in the target area.

List all the food and the drink that you consume for the next two days; don't leave anything off the list, however small the quantity. This may seem like a laborious task, but it is important that you do it, and do it accurately.

What you need to eat and drink

Separate the foods on your list into three boxes as follows:

List A	List B	List C
High Water Content Foods	**All Other Foods**	**Drinks**
1) Fruit		1) Diuretic
		a) Alcohol
2) Vegetables		b) Coffee/Tea
		2) Other
3) Salad		3) Water

Now delete the foods in List A which have been boiled, fried, grilled or baked as they will have less nutritional value. The food which remains in List A has the highest nutritional value and water content, and intake should be increased. Accordingly, intake of food under List B should be reduced.

Where possible, buy organic fruit, vegetables and salads (which most large supermarkets now stock); much traditionally grown food of this kind has suffered from the effects of modern farming techniques, destroying a great deal of its nutritional value. The body consists of between seventy and eighty per cent water, which is why we need water for our well-being. However, merely drinking water doesn't do the trick; you have to eat foods which are rich in water, that is fruit, vegetables and salad. You also have to eat them, where possible, in a natural state – uncooked.

The nutrients in our food are transported to the cells by water; similarly, the toxic waste in cells is removed by water. The water in such foods takes it to the intestine for digestion where the nutrients are removed and transported by water to the cells. Ironically, if we drink water with our meals it dilutes our digestive juices; this means we require more energy to do the same job. If we eat fruit for breakfast on its own, however, it increases our energy.

The object of a high water content diet is threefold:

1 The hair growth programme increases the movement of lymph throughout the body. By continually taking on more fluid, you literally 'flush out' your system; this removes toxins, because the body is very good at maintaining the correct fluid level, disposing of what it does not need.

2 Fruit, vegetables and salad – as well as having a high water content – also contain a high level of fibre. This improves bowel movement, and hence again flushes the system through. These foods are high in natural building blocks, and are easily digested.

3 When fruit is eaten *on its own* on an empty stomach, such as for breakfast, it passes through the stomach in fifteen to thirty minutes; from there it goes into the intestines, where it releases its sugars. It follows that because fruit takes the least amount of energy to digest, it gives your body the most in return. Fruit is primarily fructose, which the body easily converts into glucose, hence increasing energy levels rapidly. If a fruit breakfast is not substantial enough then leave twenty minutes after eating the fruit before eating additional food.

N.B. If you have advanced arthritis, this may aggravate the condition.

Your future eating habits

Try to increase your water intake, by drinking (ideally) up to 8 glasses per day. Alcohol and coffee constrict the capillaries; if taken in excess, they will undo some of the good the programme achieves. Alcohol also dehydrates the body, so compensate by drinking more water when consuming alcohol.

It is not the intention to get you to adopt strict dietary disciplines. The purpose is rather to educate you to be aware of what you are eating and drinking, and where possible and appropriate, to eat higher water content food. The energy you will gain can then be used elsewhere to combat stress, grow your hair and remove waste products from your body. As I noted at the beginning of the chapter, it is important to eat some protein (around 2oz) every day. The following foods are protein-rich: lamb, beef, pork, veal, poultry, rabbit, fish, crab, shrimp, prawns, lobster, eggs, cheese, pulses (such as lentils and chick peas) and nuts.

The task, therefore, is to keep increasing the List A food in your diet, until such time that it reaches around seventy-five per cent of what you eat. If you gradually change over, this will soon become a habit. It also requires some serious eating, so logically if we reduce our List B and D foods we should change direction without effort.

Balancing your body chemistry

A high water content diet also increases the body's alkali reserve which is crucial for good health. Many people in the UK allow their bodies to become too acidic, a contributory factor in many common diseases.

The following eating rule should help: if it has a high water content eat it and if it comes from something that once had a face, eat less of it.

Vitamins and minerals

We process and cook our food to such an extent that much of the nutritional value goes out of it. It may, therefore, be necessary to supplement your diet with extra vitamins and minerals. The following charts show you which are necessary for hair growth, where they can best be found naturally, and what the symptoms of deficiency are.

Nutrient sources

VITAMIN A	*VITAMIN B2*	*VITAMIN C*
Halibut liver oil	Yeast extract	Acerola
Liver	Dried brewer's	Cherry juice
Butter	yeast	Camupulp
Cheese	Liver	Rosehip syrup
Eggs	Wheatgerm	Blackcurrants
	Cheese	Guavas

VITAMIN E	ZINC	IODINE
Wheatgerm oil	Oysters	The iodine
Soya bean oil	Liver	content of food
Maize oil	Brewer's yeast	is meaningless,
Safflower oil	Shellfish	because the
Sunflower oil	Meat	content of the
		soil is what is
		appropriate.

Symptoms of nutrient deficiency

VITAMIN A	VITAMIN B2	VITAMIN C
Scaly skin and scalp	Hair loss	Skin haemorrages and high cholesterol

VITAMIN E
As it prevents arteriosclerosis and thrombosis and protects Vitamin A, its deficiency in relation to hair loss is apparent. It is a blood vessel dilator, and maintains healthy blood vessels.

ZINC
Hair loss

IODINE
Hair loss

Avoid vitamin 'crazes'

As you walk along the supermarket and pharmacy shelves there is a proliferation of vitamins. As I have mentioned, the way you run the body will dictate the increased/decreased demand for nutrients. In addition, certain supplements knock out the absorption of others. The best way to give your body its required amounts of the nutrients it needs is to use a Body Absorption and Nutritional Characteristic Analysis (BANCA) which identifies nutritional deficiencies. I am finding that most people with hair loss are nutritionally deficient in some way. There is no point, however, in taking supplements until you know from the BANCA report how efficiently the body is operating and where deficiencies are. (See page 111 for the information on where to get further information on the BANCA report).

Chapter 4

The Stress Response

The real problem

Let's recap a little. The causes of baldness are: poor blood supply, muscular tension, insufficient nutrients and a sluggish lymphatic system. These are separate manifestations of the same problem, but as the basic problem is a tough one to deal with quickly, you are doing scalp and neck exercises to jump-start the system. This means that you need wait no longer to grow your hair back. Behind the above causes of hair loss is the real problem: our stress response; to be precise, how often we use the stress response and how long we use it before calming the system back down again.

The problem is difficult to deal with, because our lifestyle moves at a faster, more competitive pace all the time; it is as if we continually have to run our bodies in a state of emergency. This occurred to me when I visited Tanzania and saw the pace of life of some of the local people. The pace of their lives was dictated by how fast you can travel on foot, so there was no real deadline to rush to achieve. Dinner-time was sometime in the evening! Having no electricity meant they had a lot of time to relax in the evening, allowing their bodies time to recover from the physical activity of the day. The food they ate was organic and grown locally, eaten fresh, with little processing.

It was an ideal opportunity for me to observe how although the basic 'machine' has stayed the same, we in the West have departed far from such a simple existence, forcing ourselves to sustain the incredible pace set by modern living. The problem for us is that our bodies are on full alert all the time; after a while this feels so natural that we get hooked on the high created by our own adrenalin.

So what is stress?

The term stress is used so much these days that it is difficult to pin-point what is meant by it. The tribesman could identify his source of stress very easily, because he had limited decisions to make in the day: shall I eat, shall I sleep, shall I gather wood, berries or tend my cattle? You can guess, therefore, what stress was to him – wild animals or other tribesmen attacking or stealing his cattle. From this simple lifestyle it is easy to build up a matrix of what stress is and how it affects us.

Most of us know the expression 'fight or flight' syndrome, but what happens internally, what messages do we send ourselves about what is going on?

1 Fight   – Anger
2 Flight   – Fear
3 Physical discomfort   – Pain

My tribesman, therefore, can categorize his stress very easily:

1 A lion attacks his cattle   – Anger
2 A lion threatens to attack him   – Fear
3 He cuts himself badly   – Pain

At another level he weaves a more complex set of emotions around the same basic responses. Cattle are a status symbol in this part of the world, so the same event could trigger off other emotions:

1 Obtaining the cattle can   – Aggression
make him competitive
2 A lion attacks his cattle   – Fear of loss of status
3 A lion may attack him   – Fear of personal
injury, fear for how
his family would
survive without him
4 He cuts himself badly   – Fear of infection,
being unable to
work and eat, being
unable to provide
for his family

It follows that it need not be what is going on that bothers him, but how he projects what *could* go on that arouses his adrenalin – a lion attack, for example.

In our environment, stress comes from more complex sources, so it is easier to look at distress of our mind and body to narrow the reasons down. Various events will distress us, so we have to rev up the system to deal with the extra demand or challenge. We do this by releasing adrenalin into our blood. Once the situation has been dealt with we can change back down a gear and coast along until another stressor comes along, reducing the adrenalin levels in the interim.

In our childhood stress came from being told that we could not have or do the things we wanted. Some form of authority had control over us. Adult stress is much the same, in that some authority – real or imagined – stops us having what we want, so we change up a gear. We keep changing up until we are in top gear; if our body is still distressed, we cannot go any higher and that in itself is a source of stress.

In our competitive society challenges are placed upon us from an early age – from studying hard at school and university in order to 'succeed', to forming emotional/sexual relationships. We then enter the working environment, which in itself is competitive and cut-throat. The list of what demands our time, energy and money – from mortgages to marriage – seems endless. Whole nations seem to live in this way.

Once the machine is revved up and used to living in the higher gears, it associates its achievements with living at that pace, and does not want to change back down again. The stress response is designed as a temporary response; we cannot stay in an emergency state continually without paying the price with our physical health.

Your Life Plan

Ask yourself some simple questions:

1 Is your life going the way you want it to?
2 Are you happy and content with most of it?

3 Have you fulfilled your ambitions in every department of your life?

4 Are the events in your life the result of an overall master-plan that you have consciously structured and regularly review?

5 Are you swept along by a current that seems so strong that you have to apply all your energy just to keep afloat?

Let me assure you that if you have not designed a life plan for yourself, someone else will fit you into theirs. The purpose of this book is to restore your hair growth, not to instruct you on personal management. Your overall health and happiness, however, should be of concern to you in order to obtain maximum benefit from the programme.

Write down in detail where you think you would like to be in five years' time. The exercise in itself is powerful, and highlights the areas you may wish to move away from, and those you wish to concentrate on. The following list should help, but is not definitive; it is designed to spur you into writing your own.

1 *Health* What shape do you want your hair, body, fitness, teeth, skin to be in?

2 *Relationships* How do you view your ideal relationship with partner, children, neighbours, friends, colleagues, parents.

3 *Education* What would you like to be able to do that you cannot do now:

a Play a musical instrument

b Learn another language

c What else do you want to know?

4 *Work*

a What would be your ideal job?

b How should your colleagues relate to you?

c How far would you want to travel to your workplace?

d Will you be creative in your work?

e Would you be retired or semi-retired?

5 *Financial Matters*

a How much income do you wish to have?

b What capital would you ideally wish to have?

c What sort of house would you like?

d What car would you be driving?

e Where would you go on holiday?

f What clothes would you wear?

6 *Community Service*

a How could you help your friends/family/relatives?

b How could you help in your local community?

c What knowledge could you share with others?

7 *Personal Development*

If you had to list three things about your personality that you would like to change, what would they be?

a I am shy and lack confidence

b I put things off

c I give up too easily

8 *Sport*

a What sport would you wish to learn?

b What sport do you wish to improve on?

Now go back over the list and write your answers as if anything is possible. Do not hold back – act as if you could be anyone, as if you are directing a film. The logic of this will become clearer as you proceed through this book. It is important not to become too goal-oriented, however, as failing to meet these goals may be counter-productive. Consider whether the goals you set yourself are appropriate and achievable. You should always be prepared to review them, as they may be affected by factors outside your control. Goals should be seen as guiding lights rather than fixed tracks.

Adrenalin management is awareness

As I have said, you are going to jump-start your system in order to get your hair growing while you are tackling the real issue. So we are going to take a shortcut.

Let's ignore the hundreds of chemical changes that take place when we change up through the gears, and focus on just one: vasoconstriction. Adrenalin causes the smaller, peripheral capillaries to close and transfer the blood to the 'war machine'. When this happens the skin temperature falls, as much as ten per cent when the stress is extreme.

Place your wrist against your cheek and see whether it is warm or cool; the cooler the wrist, the more vasoconstriction that is going on. (This will only work when the body temperature is settled at room temperature.) I use little plastic stress monitors which stick to the inside of the wrist and change colour depending on the temperature. These are powerfully accurate little devices as they tell you exactly what is going on in the body, not what you think is going on. (See p. 111 if you would like to order some.)

The scale on the monitors is as follows:

Blue	**Green**	**Brown**	**Black**
92°	86°–88°	82°–84°	less than 82°
Good	Quite good	Very unsettled	Bad

They also reflect the colours in between.

The object of the exercise is to quieten the body down, so releasing the vasoconstriction and returning blood to the surface capillaries.

The exercises you are already doing for your scalp have been designed to relax you and cause these capillaries to open. It is worth observing the temperature/colour of the stress monitor on your wrist before the exercises and again afterwards. If you find that you are still vasoconstricting all the time, you should turn to the relaxation techniques shown later.

You need to reduce your adrenalin flow once a day to start with, which will allow the blood to flow freely through to the scalp. Gradually, as you begin to manage your adrenalin more successfully, you will only need to do the scalp exercises and follow the relaxation techniques occasionally and hence will be feeding your hair all the time.

The important point to understand is that many physical changes are going on all over the body as you keep reaching the state required for the adrenalin release. By concentrating just on adrenalin the other changes will be controlled too. The stress response happens via a dual circuit of our nervous system and our adrenal glands. In effect our nervous system runs on automatic once we have presented information to ourselves that lets it know that we are distressed. Herein lies the secret of how to manage our adrenalin/stress response: it is how we *present* a situation and the world to ourselves that triggers the response, not how the world actually is.

The main point to remember about our physical and chemical reactions is that when we enter 'battle situations' the body fuels itself up by raising its blood sugar level. Your task is to learn to control the 'adrenalin response', gradually quietening the system down so that *you* and not other people are as much in control of your day-to-day life as possible.

Understanding your stress

As we delve deeper into stress and so begin to understand it, we can sift through the problem areas of our lives, making adjustments to ensure a more tolerable level of adrenalin.

Before starting, however, it is useful to list the areas of your life that you believe are the most problematical. Within the areas of your life that follow here, make a note each day of what is causing you problems. It may be that some things are repeated over and over again; use this as a pointer to what causes you most upset. Consider areas such as: your health, home life, relationships, working environment, education, financial position, sport, personal development (your self-esteem) and contribution to the community.

Having listed all your stressors, make a priority list of the areas you are going to work on. Resolve to reduce the level of stress from the priority areas, even if at present you cannot see how to do so.

Pain and pleasure

All of our actions come down to two very simple animal instincts: we seek pleasure and try to avoid pain. Our fight

or flight mechanism is the 'avoiding pain' part of this basic
instinct. If you did not fight you would have pain inflicted
on you; in another situation you might have pain inflicted on
you if you did not run away.

At the other end of the scale, we seek pleasure in many
ways. We may need to push ourselves a little to achieve it,
so our adrenalin system can also be triggered by pleasure-
seeking too. Our excitement at the thought of pleasure to
come can likewise raise adrenalin levels. It is possible also
for pleasurable events to raise our adrenalin levels too high,
a point often overlooked when we consider what stresses us.
A change or unexpected event can also raise our adrenalin.

In 1967, Thomas Homes and Richard Rahe studied the
health of patients over a period of two years. Following
various changes in the patients' lives, Homes and Rahe
found them to be more susceptible to illness.

From Homes and Rahe's findings the following chart has
been compiled to measure the magnitude of stress related
to change.

Change	Score	Your Score
Death of someone close	100	
Divorce/separation	73	
Injury/illness	53	
Marriage	50	
Redundancy	47	
Retirement	45	
Birth of a child	39	
Change in finances	38	
Child leaving home	29	
Completing education	27	
Change at work	20	

Moving house	16
Going on holiday	15
Christmas	12
Breaking the law	11

Count up your score of the changes that have taken place in your life over the last six months. If you score more than 50, then you are likely to be stressed by these changes. Remember, it is their compound effect that causes the stress.

I am not suggesting that you try to stop such events happening in your life; it would in any case be impossible to do so. What I propose is that you should be aware of their effect on you, paying particular attention to the fact that their compound effect means that a number of minor changes will become a serious stressor. In times of compound change, you will simply have to work much harder at relaxing your system, following a change or any source of stress.

Presenting information to yourself in a stressful way

It is often not what is actually happening to you, but how you present the information to yourself that is important. Providing we look at a situation as if there is a way out of it and ask empowering questions that lead us to new possibilities, ninety per cent of the time we will succeed in finding new solutions to old problems. If we ask questions which have within themselves implied failure, we are ninety per cent certain to fail.

I mentioned at the beginning of the book the idea of our mind sending off guided missiles which zig-zag on and off track until they strike their target. You are setting these targets by the way you tackle a problem as it arises; to be more precise, by the way in which you interpret the world around you. A question like: 'What other problems are likely to result from this event?' are 'guided missiles'. Back at control, an instruction goes something like this: 'Launch missiles 123 and 456; Andy is looking for problems associated with this event. Do not come back until you have discovered lots for him – if you cannot find any, create some.' A good question, on the other hand, can send off a beneficial missile: 'Andy is looking for a way around this, so launch missile 10. Off you go then search the entire memory bank for something or someone that may help.'

However busy you thought you were on the surface with all your problems, this subconscious level works twenty-four hours a day to solve such questions. Do not underestimate its power – for example, it is currently controlling your breathing, feeding your body its fuel, holding your muscle tension, etc. Once you have learnt to trust the method of asking good and appropriate questions, you will be astonished at how easily you find new solutions to old problems.

Personality types

Certain personality types stress themselves more than others. Meyer Friedman and Ray Roseman, two cardiologists whose research has already been mentioned (see p. 25), noted that certain personality types were more predisposed to heart attacks than others. They classified people into 'A' and 'B' type personalities and listed their characteristics.

The type 'A' was more predisposed to stress by his very personality, and therefore more prone to heart disease. I have found that he is *also* predisposed to hair loss. Check yourself against the following points:

Type 'A'

Always in a hurry
Very impatient
Does more than one thing at a time
Continually doing things; cannot rest
Aggressive
Hostile
High muscular tension
Talks fast; tries to speed up others
Tries to do things in a hurry
Competitive
Cannot accept criticism

(See Chapter 5, 'Working on your type "A" personality', pp. 86–88, to find out how you can combat these traits.)

My story may help you to focus on your own life. My health had been perfect from my teens until my early thirties. At that point stress began to wreck my body. I could then tick every one of the type 'A' personality traits. It took six whole months to get my stress dot from black to brown, and a further three months to get up to green. Now, thankfully, my dot is blue most of the time. It is not that I have a totally stress-free life – far from it. The difference lies in how I now present information to myself. My number one priority is my health and I ask the question constantly: 'Is "X" worth it for the strain it causes on my health?' Usually I find an answer which does not affect my health by turning the question round: 'How can I achieve "X" without affecting my health adversely?' Sometimes the answer is that you cannot change or have something, and in such cases I have learnt to surrender to the inevitable – without losing any sleep over it.

The following chapter, 'How to Combat Your Stress', will help you get to grips with this issue, which is at the heart of the hair growth programme.

Chapter 5

How to Combat Your Stress

Managing your life

As suggested in the previous chapter, imagine that you are the director of a film, and that the film you are directing is called *A More Balanced Life*. The size of your budget – measured in time rather than money – dictates how you construct the film. There are a number of areas your film should include:

1 Learning how to relax;
2 Getting good sleep;
3 Breathing properly;
4 Being 'present';
5 Time management;
6 Working on your type 'A' personality;
7 Learning to reward yourself;
8 Learning to worry only about what you *can* change;
9 Learning that you can change more than you think;
10 Reviewing your goals;
11 Learning to prioritize;

12 Stopping lying to yourself;
13 Planning to be stressed;
14 Including exercise in your life.

You can also *ad lib*, adding areas of your own, but do be sure to include all of the elements above. The point about this film is that you are directing it, no one else. Do not tell your friends that you are doing this, and see if they notice a change in you. In the following pages I will guide you, but you are going to have to do the rest. I have given you exercises that are going to jump-start the engine – the speed of full recovery will depend on how you direct the film. Keep your mind on the goal of restoring your hair growth.

A word of warning: it is easy to put off starting in order to finish off something else, so don't delay. Similarly it is easy to declare that you have not had difficulties in these areas of your life; try all the same to include everything I have mentioned – you might surprise yourself!

1 Learning how to relax

The first stage of relaxation is a jump-start. The following relaxation exercises are designed to shut down anyone, whatever the source of their stress. The conscious mind can only concentrate on one thing at a time, even though the type 'A' personality does not know this. Look at his desk, and you would think that he could do twenty things at once. If you doubt the wisdom of this, try counting to ten and saying the alphabet backwards at the same time! By giving the mind a relaxation exercise that keeps it busy, it is difficult for it to focus on its problems, and thus a state of relaxation is achieved.

There is an inseparable link between body posture and mental attitude. Stressful events cause the mind to fire off certain muscle groups; the reverse is also true, in that relaxing the muscles also relaxes the mind. Try to remember to check your posture for unnecessary tension periodically throughout the day. For example, when driving, check to see whether there is too much tension in between the shoulders, or that your arms are gripping the steering wheel with more force than you need to. Rotate the shoulders and soften your grip fractionally. At the traffic lights (with the handbrake on) stretch your neck muscles and scalp muscles.

When walking, slow your pace down, and practise abdominal breathing (see p. 84). Once you are abdominally breathing to a ratio of 5/20/10, breathe in, hold, and breathe out. As you do so, focus your attention on each step. Place your heel on the ground fractionally before the foot. Become aware of just how you walk. Think about all those muscles that you usually fire off automatically: how do you swing your arms? How does your head move? Do you swing from the hip, knee or both?

Everyday relaxation techniques

Level 1

First place the stress dot on your wrist (see p. 69 for more information about stress dots). Sit comfortably in a chair. Breathe out as far as you can, drawing the abdomen (stomach) in and up. Hold your breath for a couple of seconds once you have fully exhaled. Then draw a deep breath without raising your chest, allowing the abdomen to expand, and pushing it downwards as if you are pushing the air down through your backside. Again hold this position for a few seconds. Now breathe out again *slowly*, drawing the abdomen back in and up to the starting position. Repeat this exercise as slowly as possible, and take between ten to twenty breaths. However, inhale to the count of five, hold for a count of twenty and exhale for a count of ten.

I like to refer to relaxation as Levels 1 to 4. I picture myself in an elevator going down to a floor below ground. This exercise will get you to Level Minus 1. It is an easy one to do on a train journey or while waiting for someone, as you can do it without drawing too much attention to yourself.

Level 2
Relaxation exercise for five to ten minutes per day.

1 Get yourself comfortable on a bed/floor or in a chair.
2 Start off with the breathing exercise above.
3 As you complete the tenth/twentieth breath tense your lips and then relax them. As they relax, search internally for a light, tingling sensation. The more you concentrate the stronger the feeling may appear.
4 Then tense both hands and relax them. Place your attention inside the hands to find the tingling sensation.
5 Move around your entire body this way: feet, calves, thighs, stomach, arms, shoulders, neck, face, paying particular attention to the scalp muscles.
6 If you find your mind wandering back to your problems, break away from the tension/relaxation and go back to breathing. After completing three breaths you will find it easier to go back to tension/relaxation.

Level 3
If you want to go deeper you should complete the entire exercise of Level 2 very slowly, gently applying the tension/

relaxation a second time around. Do not worry if you fall asleep. Often our stress and muscular tension affects our sleeping. When we do give our bodies permission to relax they often catch up on their sleep too.

You may find that after a couple of days following the relaxation exercises you sleep better and more deeply at night.

Level 4

Relaxation tapes are a good way of taking you more deeply down into yourself. The problem with them is that when the body is in a deep state of relaxation it can take suggestions on board rather literally. These tapes are often almost hypnotic. The only way to get to know the content is to listen to the tape, by which time it is too late! I have prepared my own tapes specifically for 'hair growers' (see p. 111 for information on how to buy these tapes).

Having relaxed your body using the above techniques, the tension in your scalp should begin to subside. This will change the colour of the stress dot.

2 Getting good sleep

How much sleep do you need? Only your body knows the answer to this; depending on the time which it perceives as available, and on the adrenalin rushing through your veins, your body will adjust the length and depth of your sleep accordingly.

Sleep is the most powerful weapon you have to combat the harmful effects of stress on your body, so do not underestimate its benefits. As we spend twenty to thirty per cent of our life sleeping, it is clearly a necessity for our health and well-being.

There are two main phases of sleep: REM and non-REM sleep. REM stands for Rapid Eye Movement, where the eyes are seen to move around fast under the eyelids. It is the dreaming phase of sleep. Non-REM sleep can be broken down into three stages, by monitoring the electrical activity in the brain. You should pass from stage 1 through to stage 4 three to five times a night. It is during stage 4 sleep that the body moves about.

During the first forty-five minutes, your heart rate and blood pressure slow, and you drop down to stage 4 sleep; we descend from stage 1 to stage 4 more than once during the night. The next forty-five minutes brings you back up to stage 1, from where REM sleep is entered. During REM sleep – about twenty-five per cent of total sleep – the skeletal muscles are inhibited from movement, but blood pressure and heart rate increase. We gradually surface throughout the night into a lighter and lighter sleep.

The true purpose of sleep is as yet undefined. I favour the idea of the body using the time to clean the waste produced in the system by the nervous activity of the day. I believe that some sorting out and storing of information is also going on in the brain during sleep.

If you are deprived of either REM or non-REM sleep, when you next sleep your sleeping pattern is altered for a period of time, as if a catching up is necessary. I certainly found that when I was woken by an alarm clock to ensure I was up each morning to beat the traffic, I would crash out anywhere and everywhere while on holiday.

Working on the assumption that enough sleep at all levels is important, why can we not get to sleep when we are tired, or what stops us falling down into level 4 sleep? Adrenalin activates the arousal system in the brain, firing us up for action. The body must be still to induce sleep, or gently and rhythmically rocked – as a baby knows only too well. The body in an aroused state tosses and turns all night. This arousal keeps us from descending to the deeper levels of sleep; we awake still feeling tired, which in turn makes us perform badly. This creates more stress, more adrenalin, less sleep, more stress and so on in a vicious circle.

Darkness sends messages to the brain to sleep, so darken your bedroom as much as possible. Try gradually dimming the lights to induce sleep throughout the evening. If you live in a noisy area wear ear plugs.

Calculate how much sleep you need by adding half an hour per night for the first month. Then the next month increase this by another half an hour, and so on until you reach the optimum sleeping period suitable for you. If this is not possible during the week, add extra sleeping time at the weekends.

Do not watch films or read novels that trigger your adrenalin response. Nor should you work in bed or late at night, as this will keep your mind busy.

So far with your adrenalin management you have short-circuited the system; your body fires itself up, and you then relax it as described earlier. If you do nothing else, the relaxation exercises you have learnt, together with getting good sleep, will set you on the road to a dramatic improvement in your adrenalin management, and consequently an improvement in your overall health.

Avoid eating any food late at night. Some foods tend to wake us up, especially protein foods (meat, fish, nuts etc), sugary foods and spicy foods. Drinks can also keep you awake, such as coffee, tea, chocolate and alcohol. Too much alcohol makes us want to urinate during the night, pulling us up out of level 4. In moderation, though, it can help us sleep. Other foods like carbohydrates (bread, pasta, noodles etc), can make us drowsy.

3 Breathing properly

The abdominal breathing exercises you have learnt lower your adrenalin response. When the body is stressed, we tend to breathe fast bouts of short breaths high in the chest. By deliberately interrupting the pattern, our bodies quieten down the stress response. Do not reserve the breathing techniques just for your scalp exercises; use them whenever you get wound up. For example, I always use them when I am in a traffic jam, or when I am waiting for an appointment or standing in a queue.

4 Being 'present'

Most of our anxiety comes not from what is actually happening in our lives, but what we believe may happen, or what happened in the past that we remain unhappy about. One of your objectives should be to live as much as possible in the present, rather than looking back or projecting forward. Most of us are inclined to look to the future, instead of concentrating on the here-and-now. We worry about things that never happen – and we can also never be sure of the way our lives will unfold. Do not waste your mental energy in this way.

If you must keep replaying an old mental 'video', visualize it not as it was, but as you wish it might have been. The more detailed and explicit your visualization, including introducing sound, smell, taste and touch, the quicker your memory banks will replace the old unhappy event with the new imagined one. Before too long, it will be impossible to rerun the original version. (Of course I am not saying that genuinely traumatic events can in themselves be altered, but certainly their effect on your life can be adjusted.)

Similarly, if you are worried about a future event, run the 'video' over in your mind with everything going perfectly. Try to make yourself feel calm, strong and in control. If you cannot muster up those feelings, go back to an old memory of when you felt in control in order to help you now.

5 Time management

Much of your stress can be self-imposed by being badly organized. Some simple rules will help. Always start the day with a priority list of jobs – jobs to do, telephone calls to make, letters that need writing etc, depending on what your job is, or how you spend your time if you are unemployed. This list should be planned the day before; this will stop your mind racing with thoughts of what you have to do when you are trying to sleep. Also try to calculate how long each job will take, and do not set yourself impossible goals.

Adopt the habit of filing papers at the end of each day. Put a note in your diary as to when you intend to deal with something, whenever that will be. Once you have adopted this habit, try not to take work home; finish in your office, leaving work mentally as well as physically. Those who do this will have little problem with time management.

Some days you become inundated, and your 'to do' list is longer at the end of the day than when you started. Be positive about this; it may show how important you are, if so many people need your help! Never worry or feel guilty that you could not get it all done: the twenty-four-hour day will never get longer, and you can only do so much.

If you are trying (or expected) to do too much, explain the problem to your boss. Ask how he would deal with the situation, unless of course you are the boss – in which case it may indicate that extra help is needed, or that you should prioritize the work you do yourself.

If you seem to be always too busy for a holiday, get in the habit of allocating yourself some weeks off in advance, and put them in your diary. Also write in the odd day's holiday – and take it.

When you are due to do something, do it – never put things off. Procrastination can become a habit.

You also need to learn to say no, at least some of the time – do not expect to be able to fulfil *all* the demands other people may make of you.

6 Working on your type 'A' personality

Certain personality types stress themselves more than others. In the early days of the programme it was very clear that most of my clients were type 'A' personalities.

To begin with, you must understand that you *are* a type 'A' personality; it helps in this respect to have a close friend or partner to look at your responses to the questions on p. 75 with you. Once you can see that you do have personality traits that need to be adjusted, the following points should help you.

Aggression raises your stress level, and is in fact counter-productive. If you know what you want to achieve, and you are assertive rather than aggressive, you can get the same end result but without the negative effects on your health caused by aggression. Aggression makes the adrenal glands release hormones which create more aggression; what you need to do is break out of this vicious circle.

Another important trait to tackle is competitiveness. We are taught from a very young age that it is right to be competitive; however, a great price – in terms of your general health – can be paid for winning. It is essential to see that coming second or third – if it still gets you where you want to go – is just as valuable. Many salesmen drive themselves into serious ill health through their desire to surpass unrealistic targets.

The type 'A' personality is always rushing against the clock, with self-imposed deadlines. He therefore compensates by trying to do more than one thing at a time. This becomes so subtle that he rarely recognizes what he is doing. For a week, be aware of what you are actually doing rather than what you think you are doing, and ask your workmates or partner to comment. For example, do you: dress or shave in the car, read your post while you are on the telephone, or work on the computer while you are on the telephone? If so, this is actually the result of poor time management, and setting an unrealistic time limit on what you are doing – both of which you can change. Try deliberately slowing yourself down – walk more slowly and drive within the speed limit, for example.

You may have difficulty in relaxing. If so, turn to the sections on time management (p. 85) and learning how to relax (p. 78) which will help in this respect.

Any tendency you have towards impatience should diminish once you have mastered time management, and how to relax. Watch yourself next time you are in the queue at the post office or bank; use the breathing exercises (p. 84) to calm yourself down.

7 Learning to reward yourself

To follow the programme you may need to make many changes in your life, and take a disciplined approach about it. Above all, do not take life so seriously. Wind down and enjoy yourself more – smile and laugh more. Reward yourself on a regular basis for achieving your goals. These rewards should go with the general flow of reducing your adrenalin and growing back your hair. I use the following:

- a top-to-toe massage occasionally;
- a head massage;
- a weekend break somewhere relaxing;
- a special evening out with a partner or close friend;
- a small gift for achieving a particular goal.

Learn to love yourself as you are. You are a unique individual, and your failings in one department are made up for by the qualities you have in another. Try reflecting on your good points and achievements for a while. If you do this while you are doing the exercises as suggested, and following your new Life Plan, you will find that any changes you *do* need to make will happen naturally.

Reflect upon the successes in your life. Congratulate yourself, and become aware that the new goals you are setting are well within your grasp.

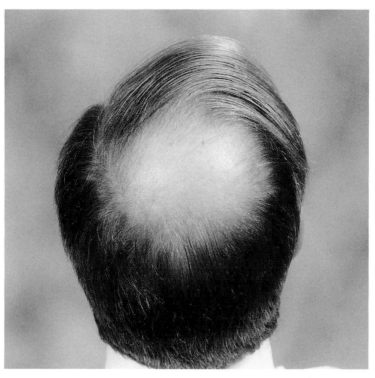

Robin Stevens
Measurement of bald spot: 60 sq cm, July 1992
Shiny bald

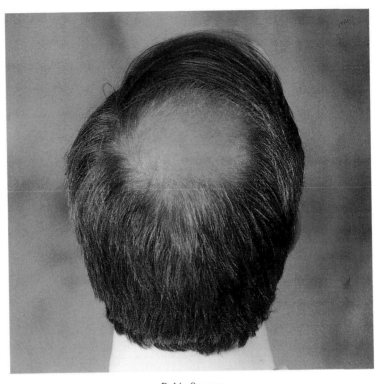

Robin Stevens
Measurement of bald spot: 36 sq cm, August 1993
Scalp tension gone

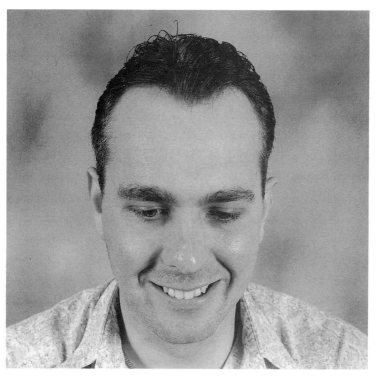

Mike Simmons
Measurements:
(a) from tip of nose to centre of hair line: 14.5cm
(b) from tip of nose to parting: 19.5 cm, October 1992
Severe receding hair line

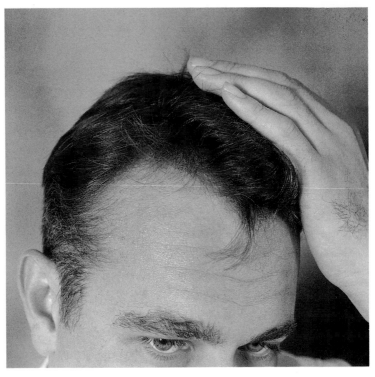

Mike Simmons
Measurements:
(a) from tip of nose to centre of hair line: 13 cm
(b) from tip of nose to parting: 17 cm, August 1993
Hair line virtually back to normal

8 Learning to worry only about what you *can* change

Worry is simply inaction by another name. Once you have an action plan, worry quietens down. The simple message is to act, not worry. Managing your time better (as on pp. 85–86) will help you deal with worry also.

If you feel that you cannot solve your problems alone, seek professional guidance; do not bottle them up inside. Just as a kettle has to release its steam, your problems will surface in your mind time and time again. Often they manifest in illness, so resolve to deal with them – never give up.

9 Learning that you can change more than you think

If I were to challenge you to improve any three areas of your life over the next five years, in competition with a five-year-old child, you would probably feel that I had gone too far. Consider the following before writing this idea off.

Children come into the world without knowing what it is about, and create their own mental maps. Those maps are well and truly sketched by the age of ten. Up until that age, the child will not have put up the barriers that we as adults have created. Adults are over-concerned about making a fool of themselves in front of others, and worry too much about what other people think of them.

Most of what we do not achieve in life is not based upon what we can or cannot achieve. It is based instead upon what we *believe* we are capable of. Young children feel that all things are possible; they have not learnt the social inhibitions that can prevent adults from achieving their full potential.

In my own case, I was very inhibited about public speaking – which I need to do in conjunction with my hair growth programme. I used to worry about coping with technical questions from doctors sceptical about the programme. Eventually I had to face my greatest fear, a very technical question. I answered not by allowing myself to get caught up in technicalities but by simply saying that the proof was in the new hair growing on so many heads. The fear I had about coping with such questions was much worse than the event itself!

Remind yourself from time to time that you can achieve more than you thought you could – don't let your fears control your actions.

10 Reviewing your goals

Unless you know where you are going and have plotted a rough journey, it is difficult to get there. Earlier you listed where you want to be in five years time. Now you need the algebra to work in your subconscious. If you know how many hours you have allocated daily to the different 'compartments' of your life and where you wish to be, your subconscious can begin to plot the right course. Remember that you are the director of the film of your life, and are plotting where you would like to be and the route you will take to achieve the aims in your Life Plan.

Do not be too hard on yourself over failure in any area; just resolve to work harder at the task in future. If one route to where you would like to be does not work or you go off course, simply try again or try a slightly different course.

Remember how the guided missile works – all feedback is positive. If you go off track you know now how not to do so in future. You have not failed; if anything you have got nearer your goal than when you started, because next time you will recognize when you are going off track.

11 Learning to prioritize

Each day has only twenty-four hours in it. I have seen many advancements in my life, but no one has found a way of stretching the day, yet! Once you accept this and realize that certain things have to be done each day you can either rush around trying to beat the clock, or just take time as it flows.

Imagine if the day only had twelve or fourteen and a half hours left after the following tasks:

	24 Hours	*24 Hours*
Sleeping	7	8
Eating	1	1.5
Travelling	0	1
Washing/dressing	0	0.5
Relaxing/hair growing	1.5	1
TOTAL	9.5	12
BALANCE	14.5	12

In that time you have to look after your health, have a family life, socialize etc. Complete the hours you intend to allocate to these areas of your life, and do not let them add up to any more than the totals shown:

Work
Exercise/sport
Family/friends
Community work
Education
Religion
Other

BALANCE	14.5	12

Looked at logically, it makes the way we rush around trying to put more hours into the day than are possible, look foolish.

If you consider that you have a quota of time available (with, say, eight working hours) then you should be very careful how you allocate them. Form the habit of prioritizing certain tasks, and work out how long each job will take (as in time management). If, as in this example, your work time quota is eight hours, but your priority list shows you need ten, it is clearly not going to be possible to do all the jobs on your priority list. Be tough on yourself, because the easiest thing in the world to do is to keep taking time from other areas of your life; this works short term, but will eventually cause you serious problems.

Review the priority list; if it is truly in order of importance, the last items will have to be moved to another day. Alternatively, you will have to delegate, if you can.

12　Stopping lying to yourself

It is always easy if things go wrong to blame others. It is much more difficult to accept your own faults. You can change yourself fairly quickly, but waste a lifetime trying to change others. Try to be aware of this fact when problems arise. Have the courage to look at yourself first and see how you could have done or arranged things differently.

You may also find that your problems develop into a pattern, where a similar thing goes wrong time and time again, for no apparent reason. When this happens you may find that you attract such problems to yourself on a subconscious level. It is often one of those guided missiles I mentioned previously, set up earlier in your life, which keeps trying to hit the wrong target.

Be straight with yourself about what you want and what only *you* can do to achieve it.

13 Planning to be stressed

There will inevitably be days or weeks when you will be stressed. Try to plan in advance what you can do to prevent your being swept along with the emotional current that will be flowing at the time. You have an action plan of how to deal with your stress. So, like a fire drill, practise what you will do when the event arises. When it then happens, you can stay calm and in control of the situation as you would with a fire drill. Obviously your personal action plan will depend on your work and family circumstances. One thing to remember, though, is that you should not be too proud to ask for help from others, help which you can arrange to give them on another occasion.

14 Including exercise in your life

As I have explained in previous chapters, you need to restore blood flow to the scalp. Any form of aerobic exercise will be beneficial to this objective.

I recommend that you gradually increase the amount of exercise you take so that eventually you are doing an optimum of twenty minutes of aerobic activity every other day. If you currently have a lifestyle that does not allow for this, try changing slowly by setting aside time for one session per week. Only increase this once you have been sticking to it each week. Choose an exercise which you really enjoy as it is then easy to include it in your daily routine. The following table is a useful guideline:

	1st qtr	2nd qtr	3rd qtr	4th qtr
Totally unfit	5 mins	10 mins	15 mins	20 mins
Reasonably fit	10 mins	15 mins	20 mins	20 mins
Super fit	30 mins	30 mins	30 mins	30 mins

These times are based on each forty-eight-hour period.

If you conscientiously and methodically set out to follow the suggestions in this chapter you will considerably reduce – if not eliminate – your stress.

Chapter 6

People on the Programme

Having discovered why baldness occurs and having helped a number of people overcome it, I was taken aback that no one would believe it was so simple. How could I prove the success of the programme? I considered the way that drug companies established their proof, by means of clinical trials. A large number of people would be told they were using a drug known to help cure baldness. Some would be given the drug and others a placebo; many weeks into the trial the placebo would be switched to the actual drug. It is because neither the doctor administering the drug nor the patient knows whether or not the drug or a placebo is being taken that the trials are known as double blinds. As many drugs have side effects, part of any trial involves full medical tests, in order to detect any problems.

My methods involved no drugs, however. It is also rather difficult to have half the group invert and do muscle tension exercises as they learn to control their stress and learn to relax, and the rest not, but think they were! In fact my control group consisted of one hundred men selected during 1992, all of whom knew what they were doing and why.

I could compare them against the other eight million British men who were doing nothing, and not re-growing their hair. After six months, ninety-seven per cent of the first hundred people on the programme were growing hair at a reasonable rate.

Eventually I asked a mathematician to devise an evaluation report. He specializes in preparing clinical trials for drug companies and favoured actually counting the hairs grown. As this was not a medical product, we decided to train hairdressers to do the count. This turned out to be a tougher assignment than we imagined. Our problem was that so much new hair was coming through after six months that it was not only boring counting thousands of hairs but the head was literally covered in minute green felt tip ticks! Clearly those on the programme were growing too much hair to count it. If we were growing a handful of hairs it would be easy, but we had people with complete coverings of previously bald spots. Here we were growing hair at a rate that a non-expert could see from a distance let alone need to count, so we have decided to let the proof speak for itself.

Personal success stories

The best thing about this programme is that the people on it are so happy to be growing their hair back. I have now seen over 200 people who are re-growing their hair. The following four hair participants can speak for themselves, with their personal success stories. (To understand the measurements given, see the section of this chapter on recording your progress, pp. 102–103.)

Case History 1

Name: David Clark-Wilson   **Age:** 40
Baldness pattern: Bald Crown (Friar Tuck)

Andy told me about his new cure for baldness in November 1991. I didn't believe him, although eventually I said I'd do the programme just to prove him wrong. Six weeks later I was already growing new hair and had to go back and apologize for my lack of faith.

My father was a doctor, who had lost virtually all his hair by the age of twenty-three. With my own back-ground as a mathematics scholar, I was able to look at the programme logically; nobody I have spoken to can explain why I should stop growing hair having learnt how to grow it, and it has carried on growing ever since, increasing in strength.

Weaknesses

1 I still have problems with stress dot monitor colour, and vasoconstriction.
2 I didn't understand the importance of scalp tension initially, and thought it was all about inversion.

Side benefits

1 Lost about 21 lb in weight.
2 Improved skin condition (no longer dry).
3 Eliminated sore throats.
4 General all round improvement in health, especially ears, nose, throat.

Start date: 22 March 1992
Initial measurement: 102 sq cm
Latest measurement Date: 13 November 1993
Latest measurement: 20 sq cm

Case History 2

Name: Robin Stevens   **Age:** 55
Baldness pattern: Receding, and bald crown
It took me just thirty minutes to get involved in the programme, having lost hair at the crown and the temples
over a period of seven years. It was really my daughter's
wedding which made me think about the lack of hair on my
crown, when the video showed up my bald pate. It was
horrible.

I have now been on the programme for eleven months,
and the results are remarkable.

Weaknesses
   1 Work stress – building industry!

Side benefits
   1 Improved sex life.
   2 Removal of tension from my neck, back and shoulders.
   3 Improved sleeping.

Start date: July 1992
Initial measurement: 60 sq cm
Latest measurement Date: July 1993
Latest measurement: 36 sq cm

Case History 3

Name: Steve Coe   **Age:** 32
Baldness pattern: Receding and thinning on crown
I was much more interested in the stress part of the programme than hair growth itself. I followed the programme without using the shampoo to see what happened. I grew hair more slowly than other people, and followed the programme more diligently after three months.

I am now most impressed with the general health aspects of the programme, and have improved the quality of my life over the last year.

Weaknesses
1 I took a while to address my stress.
2 I didn't treat the dietary part of the programme seriously, initially.

Side benefits
1 Now that my stress is under control I feel more relaxed.
2 Improvement in general complexion.
3 Reduction in neck and shoulder tension.

Start date: July 1992
Initial measurement (centre): 17 cm
Initial measurement (parting): 21.5 cm
Latest measurement Date: August 1993
Latest measurement (centre): 12 cm
Latest measurement (parting): 16 cm

Case History 4

Name: Mike Simmons   **Age:** 34
Baldness pattern: Receding

I was very worried about losing my hair, which had been receding from the front for about six years. I loved the programme from the start, and started to grow hair within the first four weeks.

Being a motor cycle courier I get quite stressed driving through London traffic; following the rules for reducing stress has helped me a lot.

Weaknesses

1 My diet is not quite good enough.

Side benefits

1 I am generally more relaxed.
2 My sleep has improved dramatically.
3 My neck and shoulder tension has gone.

Start date: September 1992
Initial measurement (centre): 14.5 cm
Initial measurement (parting): 19.5 cm
Latest measurement Date: July 1993
Latest measurement (centre): 13 cm
Latest measurement (parting): 17.5 cm

Programme trial results

The first hair-growers on the programme have been photographed from the front, the side and the back. More importantly, they have been measured to determine their baldness area.

The results on the first forty hair-growers, of which twenty-six had receding hair lines and eighteen had bald areas on the crown (four had both), showed the following:

Frontal hair growth

Sample size: 26
Minimum period on programme: 6 months
Average growth per month (centre): 2.2 mm
Average growth per month (parting): 1.9 mm
Least growth (centre): 2 cm
Least growth (parting): 1.5 cm
Most growth (centre): 5 cm
Most growth (parting): 5.5 cm

Growth on the crown

Sample size: 18
Minimum period on the programme: 6 months
Average growth on the crown: 3.76 sq cm
Least growth: 8 sq cm
Most growth: 79 sq cm

Recording your progress

Your first task is to identify your baldness pattern as closely as you can from the following.

1 Diffuse (thinning all over)
2 Receding fractionally at temples
3 Advanced thinning at temples
4 Fully advanced at temples, with small circle around the front
5 Thinning crown
6 Advanced thinning crown
7 Thinning at the crown and receding
8 Advanced baldness over the top
9 High sides, but little hair on top
10 Full baldness

You then need to take whichever of the following measurements are applicable to you. Preferably ask a friend – one who will not laugh at you – to do the measuring. Accuracy is important.

Measure from the tip of your nose to the front of your hairline in the middle of your eyes. Note the measurement here: (A). (Out of interest, if you do Exercise C on p. 46 you will see that your hairline should coincide with the ridge created by the exercise.)

Now measure from the tip of your nose to the hairline's furthest point back, to the left and right, above the eyes. Note these measurements here: Left: (B1); right: (B2).

Now mark out the centre point of the balding crown by running the measuring tape from the tip of your nose to the nape of your neck. Look along the tape for where the baldness starts and note the measurement: (C1); then note where it ends: (C2). If it is not a defined line, note back to where the hair is thickest: (C2 − C1 = LENGTH).

Run the tape from the top of the right ear to the top of the left over the centre point and note the point at which there is a defined hairline either side: Left: ——(D1); right: ——(D2) (D2 − D1 = WIDTH).

To tell you the size of the overall baldness patch, do the following calculation: Πr^2 where r = (width + length) ÷ 4. (See example, below).

This test, however, cannot be one hundred per cent accurate.

It is important, having done the initial measurements above, that you fill in the following charts at the regular intervals suggested. Do not get down-hearted if you seem to make little progress at first − it will happen in time. I am always very pleased when someone beats our fastest hair growth record. Do send me copies of your records from time to time to show me how you are doing (see p. 111 for an address).

EXAMPLE:

Width	= 10 cm
Length	= 12 cm
r	= $\dfrac{22}{4}$
	= 5.5
Bald area	= 3.142 × 5.5 × 5.5 = 95 sq cm.

Initial Assessment (Pre-Treatment)

Name:
Age:
Height:
Weight:
Duration of Hair Loss:
History of Baldness
Was your mother's brother bald at age 50?:
Was your father bald at age 50?:
Was your father's brother bald at age 50?:
Do you wear a hat in your occupation?:
Is there tension in the scalp?: Severe   Mild   Negligible
Colour of stress dot at normal room temperature:

Measurements
Front
(a) Distance from tip of nose to front to hairline: ____(A)
(b) Distance from tip of nose to left and right parting:
____(B1); ____(B2)

Bald Area (Crown)
(c) Distance from tip of nose to where baldness starts and
ends: ____(C1); ____(C2)
(d) Distance from ear to ear where baldness starts and
ends: ____(D1); ____(D2)

LENGTH = C2 − C1   LENGTH =
WIDTH = D2 − D1   WIDTH =
R = (LENGTH + WIDTH) ÷ 4   R =
BALD AREA = 3.142 × R × R   BALD AREA =

Signature:............................. **Date:**...............
Witness: .... **Date:**...............

Follow-up Assessment (3 Months)

Name:
Age:
Height:
Weight:
Duration of Hair Loss:

Improvements

What improvements have you experienced since your last assessment? e.g. weight loss, reduced back problems, stopped taking certain drugs, fewer headaches, improved sleeping, etc.

1)
2)
3)
4)

Is there tension in the scalp?: Severe;   Mild;   Negligible
Colour of stress dot at room temperature:

Measurements

Front

(a) Distance from tip of nose to front to hairline: ＿＿＿(A)
(b) Distance from tip of nose to left and right parting:
＿＿＿(B1); ＿＿＿(B2)

Bald Area (Crown)

(c) Distance from tip of nose to where baldness starts and ends: ＿＿＿(C1); ＿＿＿(C2)
(d) Distance from ear to ear where baldness starts and ends: ＿＿＿(D1); ＿＿＿(D2)

LENGTH = C2 − C1   LENGTH =
WIDTH = D2 − D1   WIDTH =
R = (LENGTH + WIDTH) ÷ 4   R =
BALD AREA = 3.142 × R × R   BALD AREA =

Signature:............................. **Date**: ....
Witness: .... **Date**: ....

Follow-up Assessment (6 Months)

Name:
Age:
Height:
Weight:
Duration of Hair Loss:
Improvements
What improvements have you experienced since your last
assessment? e.g. weight loss, reduced back problems, stopped
taking certain drugs, fewer headaches, improved sleeping, etc.
1)
2)
3)
4)
Is there tension in the scalp?: Severe;   Mild;   Negligible
Colour of stress dot at room temperature:

Measurements
Front
(a) Distance from tip of nose to front to hairline: ＿＿(A)
(b) Distance from tip of nose to left and right parting:
＿＿(B1); ＿＿(B2)

Bald Area (Crown)
(c) Distance from tip of nose to where baldness starts and
ends: ＿＿(C1); ＿＿(C2)
(d) Distance from ear to ear where baldness starts and
ends: ＿＿(D1); ＿＿(D2)

LENGTH = C2 − C1   LENGTH =
WIDTH = D2 − D1   WIDTH =
R = (LENGTH + WIDTH) ÷ 4   R =
BALD AREA = 3.142 × R × R   BALD AREA =

Signature:............................. **Date:**...............
Witness: .... **Date:**...............

Follow-up Assessment (9 Months)

Name:
Age:
Height:
Weight:
Duration of Hair Loss:
Improvements
What improvements have you experienced since your last
assessment? e.g. weight loss, reduced back problems, stopped
taking certain drugs, fewer headaches, improved sleeping, etc.
1)
2)
3)
4)
Is there tension in the scalp?: Severe;   Mild;   Negligible
Colour of stress dot at room temperature:

Measurements
Front
(a) Distance from tip of nose to front to hairline: _____ (A)
(b) Distance from tip of nose to left and right parting:
_____ (B1); _____ (B2)

Bald Area (Crown)
(c) Distance from tip of nose to where baldness starts and
ends: _____ (C1); _____ (C2)
(d) Distance from ear to ear where baldness starts and
ends: _____ (D1); _____ (D2)

LENGTH = C2 − C1	LENGTH =
WIDTH = D2 − D1	WIDTH =
R = (LENGTH + WIDTH) ÷ 4	R =
BALD AREA = 3.142 × R × R	BALD AREA =

Signature:..............................   **Date:** ....
Witness: ....   **Date:** ....

Follow-up Assessment (12 Months)

Name:
Age:
Height:
Weight:
Duration of Hair Loss:
Improvements
What improvements have you experienced since your last assessment? e.g. weight loss, reduced back problems, stopped taking certain drugs, fewer headaches, improved sleeping, etc.
1)
2)
3)
4)
Is there tension in the scalp?: Severe;   Mild;   Negligible
Colour of stress dot at room temperature:

Measurements
Front
(a) Distance from tip of nose to front to hairline: ____(A)
(b) Distance from tip of nose to left and right parting:
____(B1); ____(B2)

Bald Area (Crown)
(c) Distance from tip of nose to where baldness starts and ends: ____(C1); ____(C2)
(d) Distance from ear to ear where baldness starts and ends: ____(D1); ____(D2)

LENGTH = C2 − C1   LENGTH =
WIDTH = D2 − D1   WIDTH =
R = (LENGTH + WIDTH) ÷ 4   R =
BALD AREA = 3.142 × R × R   BALD AREA =

 Signature:.............................. **Date:**................
 Witness: .... **Date:**................

Conclusion

To recap, on the evidence so far, virtually anyone who wants to regrow their hair can do so by following the programme detailed in this book.

The programme is called S.I.D.E.S., standing for Stress management, Inversion, Diet (high water content), Exercise and Shampoo. The diligence with which you follow the programme will determine the results you achieve.

The reason the programme works is precisely because it addresses the fundamental causes of baldness, which can be tested in your own experience. Only you can re-grow your own hair; what I can do is provide the means, point you in the right direction, and give you the support of other hair growers. Good Luck!

Helpful reading

A-Z of the Human Body, Reader's Digest, 1987

Adragna, Solomon Schmidt, *Human Anatomy and Physiology*, Saunders/Harcourt Brace Jovanovich, 1990

Andreas, Steve and Andrews, Connirae, *Change Your Mind and Keep the Change*, Real People Press, 1987

Fisk, Dr J. W., *Your Painful Neck and Back*, Arrow Books, 1987

Grinder, John and Bandler, Richard – complete works

Hanson, Dr Peter, *The Joy of Stress*, Pan Books, 1985

Hart, Dr Archibald D., *The Hidden Link Between Adrenalin and Stress*, Word Publishing, 1986

Kaley, Jay, *Uncommon Therapy*, Norton, 1986

Kenton, Leslie and Susannah, *Raw Energy*, Arrow Books, 1984

Long, Barry, *Stillness is the Way*, The Barry Long Foundation, 1983

Maltz, Maxwell, *Psychocybernetics*, Prentice Hall, 1960

Mervyn, Leonard, *Thorson's Complete Guide to Vitamins and Minerals*, Thorsons, 1986

Moir, Anne and Jessel, David, *Brain Sex*, Mandarin, 1989

Openshaw, Florence, *Advanced Hairdressing Science*, Longman Scientific and Technical, 1981

Robbins, Anthony – complete works

Product information

Should you wish to know more about the following products mentioned in the book a price list can be forwarded to you.

Hair growth programme

Health awareness programme

Inverter

Stress management manual

Stress monitors

Stress tapes

Shampoo

Hair growers' meetings

Hair growers' news

BANCA

Contact us at: Natural Hair Products Ltd
                The Hook
                Cedar Road
                Woking
                Surrey GU22 0JJ

                TEL: (0483) 725702

Acknowledgements

I would like to express my thanks to the following people, who have kindly contributed to making the hair growth programme successful, and to expanding my knowledge in many directions: David Clark-Wilson and his wife Judy; John Sarchet; Dr Sanjay Chaudhuri; Chris Pick, clinical nutritionist; chiropractor Giles Courtis; Andrew Nichols of Stress Check Ltd; psychologist and hypnotist Alex Needham; and Atul & Dilip. I would also like to thank all the distributors of Natural Hair Products Ltd, and all the hair growers on the programme. And finally, a special thank you to my family for their patience while I was researching this book.

Index

If you have enjoyed this book, you may also be interested in the following titles published by Vermilion:

The Allergy Survival Guide	: £10.99
Beat PMT Through Diet	: £ 6.99
Beat PMT Cookbook	: £ 6.99
Beat Sugar Craving	: £ 6.99
How to Stop Smoking	: £ 5.99
Getting Sober and Loving It	: £ 6.99
Evening Primrose Oil	: £ 6.99
Hormone Replacement Therapy	: £ 6.99
The Migraine Handbook	: £ 6.99
The Wheat and Gluten-Free Cookbook	: £ 8.99
Hypno Health	: £ 6.99
Memory Power	: £ 6.99
Lyn Marshall's Instant Stress Cure	: £ 7.99
Raw Energy	: £ 6.99

To obtain your copy, simply telephone Murlyn Services on
0279 427203

You may pay by cheque/postal order/VISA and should allow 28 days for delivery. Postage and packing is free.